The health and social effects of nonmedical cannabis use

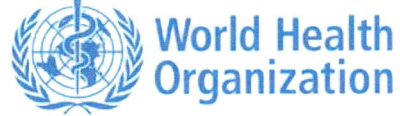

WHO Library Cataloguing-in-Publication Data

The health and social effects of nonmedical cannabis use.

1.Cannabis – adverse effects. 2.Marijuana Smoking. 3.Marijuana Abuse. I.World Health Organization.

ISBN 978 92 4 151024 0 (NLM classification: WM 276)

© **World Health Organization 2016**

All rights reserved. Publications of the World Health Organization are available on the WHO website (www.who.int) or can be purchased from WHO Press, World Health Organization, 20 Avenue Appia, 1211 Geneva 27, Switzerland (tel.: +41 22 791 3264; fax: +41 22 791 4857; e-mail: bookorders@who.int).

Requests for permission to reproduce or translate WHO publications –whether for sale or for non-commercial distribution– should be addressed to WHO Press through the WHO website (www.who.int/about/licensing/copyright_form/en/index.html).

The designations employed and the presentation of the material in this publication do not imply the expression of any opinion whatsoever on the part of the World Health Organization concerning the legal status of any country, territory, city or area or of its authorities, or concerning the delimitation of its frontiers or boundaries. Dotted and dashed lines on maps represent approximate border lines for which there may not yet be full agreement.

The mention of specific companies or of certain manufacturers' products does not imply that they are endorsed or recommended by the World Health Organization in preference to others of a similar nature that are not mentioned. Errors and omissions excepted, the names of proprietary products are distinguished by initial capital letters.

All reasonable precautions have been taken by the World Health Organization to verify the information contained in this publication. However, the published material is being distributed without warranty of any kind, either expressed or implied. The responsibility for the interpretation and use of the material lies with the reader. In no event shall the World Health Organization be liable for damages arising from its use.

Design and layout: L'iv Com Sarl
Printed by the WHO Document Production Services, Geneva, Switzerland

Contents

FOREWORD 6
ACKNOWLEDGEMENTS 7
1. Introduction 9
2. Cannabis substance profile and its health impact 10
    2.1 What do we know? 10
    2.1.1 Cannabis, cannabinoids, cannabis-use disorders 10
    2.1.2 Cannabis preparations and mode of administration 11
    2.1.3 Changes in cannabis potency 12
    2.1.4 Risk and protective factors 13
    2.1.5 Short-term health effects of cannabis use 15
    2.1.6 Long-term health effects of cannabis use 17
    2.1.7 Approach to making causal inferences 17
3. Epidemiology of cannabis use, disorders and treatment 19
    3.1 What do we know? 19
    3.1.1 Prevalence of cannabis use 19
    3.1.1.1 Global and regional data 19
    3.1.1.2 Country examples 20
    3.1.2 Prevalence of cannabis-use disorders 22
    3.1.3 Treatment trends 23
    3.1.4 Areas that require more research 25
4. Neurobiology of cannabis use 26
    4.1 What do we know? 26
    4.1.1 The psychoactive components and neurobiology of cannabis use 26
    4.1.2 Neurobiology of long-term cannabis use 27
    4.1.3 Neurobiology of prenatal cannabis exposure 28
    4.1.4 Neurobiology of cannabis effects in adolescence 29
    4.1.5 Modifiers of risk: the interplay between genetics and environment 30
    4.1.6 Areas that require more research 30
5. Short-term effects of cannabis 31
    5.1 What do we know? 31
    5.1.1 Cognition and coordination 31

5.1.2 Anxiety and psychotic symptoms 32

5.1.3 Acute toxicity 32

5.1.4 Acute cardiovascular effects 32

5.1.5 Acute effects on lungs and airways 32

5.1.6 Traffic injuries and fatalities 33

5.1.7 Other injury (not related to driving) 35

5.1.8 Cannabis and the workplace 35

5.1.9 Areas that require more research 35

6. Mental health and psychosocial outcomes of long-term cannabis use 36

6.1 What do we know? 36

6.1.1 Long-term cannabis use and dependence 37

6.1.2 Long-term cannabis use and cognitive function 38

6.1.3 Long-term psychosocial consequences of adolescent cannabis use 39

6.1.3.1 Social and educational outcomes 39

6.1.3.2 Other illicit drug use 40

6.1.3.3 Tobacco and alcohol use 41

6.1.4 Psychosis and schizophrenia 41

6.1.5 Other mental disorders 43

6.1.6 Suicide risk, ideation and attempts 44

6.1.7 Suicide mortality 45

6.1.8 Areas that require more research 46

7. Long-term cannabis use and noncommunicable diseases 47

7.1 What do we know? 47

7.1.1 Respiratory diseases 47

7.1.1.1 Chronic bronchitis 47

7.1.1.2 Chronic obstructive pulmonary disease 47

7.1.1.3 Other respiratory diseases 48

7.1.2 Cardiovascular diseases 48

7.1.2.1 Stroke 50

7.1.3 Cancer 51

7.1.3.1 Upper aerodigestive tract cancers 51

7.1.3.2 Respiratory cancers 51

7.1.3.3 Testicular cancer 52

7.1.3.4 Other cancers 52

7.1.4 Areas that require more research 53

8. Prevention and treatment 54
8.1 What do we know? 54
8.1.1 Prevention of cannabis use 54
8.1.1.1 Interventions targeting families 54
8.1.1.2 Interventions in school settings 55
8.1.1.3 Interventions targeting vulnerable youth 55
8.1.2 Treatment of disorders due to cannabis use 55
8.1.2.1 Natural history of cannabis-use disorders 55
8.1.2.2 Therapies for cannabis-use disorders 56
8.1.2.3 Management of acute cannabis intoxication and cannabis withdrawal 57
8.1.2.4 Relapse prevention 57
8.1.3 Areas that require more research 57

9. Conclusions 59
9.1 What do we know? 59
9.1.1 What do we know about the neurobiology of cannabis use? 59
9.1.2 What we know about the epidemiology of cannabis use and cannabis dependence? 59
9.1.3 What do we know about the short-term effects of cannabis use? 60
9.1.4 What do we know about the long-term effects of regular cannabis use? 60
9.1.5 What do we know about prevention and treatment? 61
9.2 Priority areas for future research 61
9.2.1 Substance content and prevalence 62
9.2.2 Neurobiology of cannabis use 62
9.2.3 Health consequences 62
9.2.4 Social costs 63
9.2.5 Prevention 63
9.2.6 Treatment 63

References 64

Foreword

Cannabis is globally the most commonly used psychoactive substance under international control. In 2013, an estimated 181.8 million people aged 15-64 years used cannabis for nonmedical purposes globally (UNODC, 2015). There is an increasing demand for treatment for cannabis-use disorders and associated health conditions in high- and middle-income countries.

Almost 20 years have passed since the World Health Organization (WHO) published a report on the health consequences of cannabis use. Since then there has been significant research on the effects of cannabis use on health. I am therefore pleased to present this update on the health and social consequences of nonmedical cannabis use, with a special focus on the effects on young people and on long-term frequent use. This report focuses on nonmedical use of cannabis, building on contributions from a broad range of experts and researchers from different parts of the world. It aims to present current knowledge on the impact of nonmedical cannabis use on health, from its impact on brain development to its role in respiratory diseases.

The potential medical utility of cannabis - including the pharmacology, toxicology and possible therapeutic applications of the cannabis plant - is outside the scope of this report.

I hope that Member States, institutions and organizations will be able to make use of this report when prioritizing areas for future international research on the health and social consequences of nonmedical cannabis use.

Dr Shekhar Saxena
Director
Department of Mental Health and Substance Abuse

ACKNOWLEDGEMENTS

The report was prepared by the Management of Substance Abuse (MSB) unit in the Department of Mental Health and Substance Abuse (MSD) of the World Health Organization (WHO), Geneva, Switzerland.

Executive editors: Wayne Hall, Maria Renström and Vladimir Poznyak.

The WHO staff involved in production of this document, developed under the overall guidance of Shekhar Saxena, Director, Department of Mental Health and Substance Abuse, were: Vladimir Poznyak, Maria Renström, Elise Gehring, Dag Rekve and Nicolas Clark. The report benefited from technical inputs to all chapters by Lauren Chidsey in her capacity as a consultant, Dr Meleckidzedeck Khayesi, Department of Management NCDs, Disability, Violence & Injury Prevention (NVI), Dr Eda Lopato, Department of Essential Medicines and Health Products (EMP) and Dr Lars Moller, WHO Regional Office for Europe.

WHO wishes to acknowledge the particular contribution of Wayne Hall, Centre for Youth Substance Abuse Research, Australia, as the main writer and editor of this document. Furthermore, special thanks are due to the members of the drafting group, namely: Louisa Degenhardt, National Drug and Alcohol Research Centre (NDARC), Australia; Jurgen Rehm, Centre for Addiction and Mental Health (CAMH), Canada; and Amy Porath-Waller, Canadian Centre on Substance Abuse (CCSA), Canada.

WHO would like to acknowledge the contributions made by the following individuals to the development of this document: Peter Allebeck, Karolinska Institute, Sweden; Courtney L Bagge, University of Mississippi Medical Center, USA; Ruben Baler, National Institute on Drug Abuse (NIDA), USA; Vivek Benegal, National Institute of Mental Health and Neurosciences, India; Guilherme Borges, Institute of Psychiatry, Mexico; Bruna Brands, University of Toronto, Canada; Paul Dargan, Guy's and St. Thomas' NHS Foundation Trust, United Kingdom; Marica Ferri, European Monitoring Centre for Drugs and Drug Addiction (EMCDDA); Valerie Wolff Galani, University Hospital of Strasbourg, France; Gilberto Gerra, United Nations Office on Drugs and Crime (UNODC); Paul Griffiths, European Monitoring Centre for Drugs and Drug Addiction (EMCDDA); Hongxing Hu, Xinjiang Medical University, China; Carlos Ibanez Pina, University of Chile, Chile; Emilie Jouanjus, University of Toulouse, France; Bertha K Madras, Harvard Medical School, USA; David Ndetei, Africa Mental Health Foundation, Kenya; Rajat Ray, Himalayan Institute of Medical Sciences, India; Jallal Toufiq, Ar-razi University Psychiatric Hospital and the National Center on Drug Abuse Prevention, Treatment and Research, Morocco; Roy Robertson, University of Edinburgh, United Kingdom; Camila Silveira, Institute of Psychiatry, University of São Paulo Medical School, Brazil; Kurt Straif, International Agency for Research on Cancer (IARC); Donald Tashkin, David Geffen School of Medicine at UCLA, USA; Nora Volkow, National Institute on Drug Abuse (NIDA), USA.

David Bramley edited the report with the help of Lauren Chidsey, and Irène R. Lengui was responsible for the graphic design and layout.

Administrative support was provided by Divina Maramba.

WHO interns who contributed to the report include: Enying Gong, Cesar Leos-Toro, Sharon Lee and Sergio Scro.

WHO gratefully acknowledges the financial and organizational support provided to this project by the Ministry of Health and Social Affairs, Sweden.

This publication contains the collective views of an international group of experts, and does not necessarily represent the decisions or the stated policy of the World Health Organization.

1. Introduction

Cannabis is globally the most commonly used psychoactive substance under international control. In 2013, an estimated 181.8 million people aged 15–64 years used cannabis for nonmedical purposes globally (uncertainty estimates 128.5–232.1 million) (UNODC, 2015). There is an increasing demand for treatment for cannabis use disorders and associated health conditions in high- and middle-income countries, and there has been increased attention to the public health impacts of cannabis use and related disorders in international policy dialogues. All this added up to the decision to publish this update report on the health and social effects of nonmedical use of cannabis.

In 1995 the World Health Organization (WHO) convened a meeting of experts on cannabis that led to the development of a report on the health consequences of cannabis use (WHO, 1997). Since then there has been significant research on the effects of cannabis use on health.

WHO (through its Department of Mental Health and Substance Abuse) organized an expert meeting on 21–23 April 2015 to review and summarize the available knowledge on the effects of nonmedical cannabis use on health and psychosocial functioning. The meeting was hosted by the Swedish Ministry of Health and Social Affairs. The purpose of the meeting was to review the latest evidence of the impact of nonmedical cannabis use on health, which is defined by WHO as a state of complete physical, mental and social well-being and not merely the absence of disease or infirmity.[1] The meeting also addressed health system responses to cannabis-use disorders and other health conditions caused by or associated with nonmedical cannabis use. It identified priorities for international research in these areas. The medical use of cannabis and cannabinoids was outside the scope of the meeting.

The meeting was attended by experts from academia, research institutions, international organizations, national health agencies. Prior to the meeting, experts were invited to produce a series of detailed background papers on the topics to be considered. These papers informed the discussions at the meeting and the meeting report that was subsequently circulated to all participating experts. A small drafting group (consisting of Professor Wayne Hall, Professor Louisa Degenhardt, Professor Jürgen Rehm, Dr Amy Porath-Waller, Ms Maria Renström and Ms Lauren Chidsey) was formed to develop a draft document that formed the basis for this publication. The draft was circulated to meeting participants and external experts for review.

This publication builds on contributions from a broad range of experts and researchers from different parts of the world. It aims to present the current knowledge on the impact of nonmedical cannabis use on health. In the process of finalizing the current report, consideration was given to the update on cannabis and cannabis resin (Madras, 2015)

---

[1] Preamble to the Constitution of the World Health Organization which was adopted by the International Health Conference held in New York from 19 June to 22 July 1946, signed on 22 July 1946 by the representatives of 61 States (Off. Rec. Wld Hlth Org. 2:100), and entered into force on 7 April 1948. Amendments adopted by the Twenty-sixth, Twenty-ninth, Thirty-ninth and Fifty-first World Health Assemblies (resolutions WHA26.37, WHA29.38, WHA39.6 and WHA51.23) came into force on 3 February 1977, 20 January 1984, 11 July 1994 and 15 September 2005 respectively and are incorporated in the present text.

commissioned by the Secretariat of the WHO Expert Committee on Drug Dependence and presented to the thirty-seventh meeting of that Expert Committee in November 2015 (WHO, 2015).

2. Cannabis substance profile and its health impact

2.1 What do we know?

2.1.1 Cannabis, cannabinoids, cannabis-use disorders

Cannabis. A generic term used to denote the several psychoactive preparations of the cannabis plant. Cannabis is the preferred designation of the plant *Cannabis sativa*, *Cannabis indica* and, of minor significance, *Cannabis ruderalis* (Gloss, 2015). Cannabis resin means "separated resin", whether crude or purified, obtained from the cannabis plant.

In this report the term "cannabis" will be used instead of marijuana or other names indigenous to local cultures. The discussion of the health and social consequences of cannabis use is limited to the nonmedical use of the cannabis plant.

Cannabinoids: Cannabinoids are a class of diverse chemical compounds that act on cannabinoid receptors in cells that modulate neurotransmitter release in the brain. The composition, bioavailability, pharmacokinetics and pharmacodynamics of botanical cannabis differ from those of extracts of purified individual cannabinoids. Cannabinoids are basically derived from three sources: (a) phytocannabinoids are cannabinoid compounds produced by plants *Cannabis sativa* or *Cannabis indica*; (b) endocannabinoids are neurotransmitters produced in the brain or in peripheral tissues, and act on cannabinoid receptors; and (c) synthetic cannabinoids, synthesized in the laboratory, are structurally analogous to phytocannabinoids or endocannabinoids and act by similar biological mechanisms. Cannabinoids are sometimes used therapeutically (e.g. for management of spasticity in multiple sclerosis or nausea in the process of cancer chemotherapy). Discussion of the health impact of the illicit use of synthetic cannabinoids is beyond the scope of this document.

Cannabis-use disorders: Cannabis-use disorders refer to a spectrum of clinically relevant conditions and are defined via psychological, social and physiological criteria to document adverse consequences, loss of control over use, and withdrawal symptoms. Cannabis-use disorders are defined in the *Diagnostic and statistical manual of mental disorders* (DSM-5; APA, 2013) and in the *International statistical classification of diseases and related health problems* (ICD-10; WHO, 1992). ICD-10 distinguishes between harmful and dependent use of cannabis, while in DSM-5 cannabis-use disorders are classified by the severity of health impairments into mild, moderate and severe disorders. Both classifications also describe a specific cannabis withdrawal syndrome which can occur within 24 hours of consumption. For cannabis withdrawal syndrome to be diagnosed, the person must report at least two mental symptoms (e.g. irritability, restlessness, anxiety, depression, aggressiveness, loss of appetite, sleep disturbances) and at least one physical symptom (e.g. pain, shivering, sweating, elevated body temperature, chills). These symptoms are most intense in the first week of abstinence but can persist for as long as a month (Hoch et al., 2015; Budney & Hughes, 2006).

2.1.2 Cannabis preparations and mode of administration

Cannabis preparations are usually obtained from the female *Cannabis sativa* plant. The plant contains at least 750 chemicals and some 104 different cannabinoids (Radwan et al., 2015; Izzo et al., 2009). The principal cannabinoids in the cannabis plant include delta-9-tetrahydrocannabinol (THC), cannabidiol (CBD), and cannabinol (CBN). THC is the primary psychoactive compound, with CBD, a non-psychoactive compound, ranking as the second cannabinoid. Generally, THC is found at higher concentrations than CBD. The known chemical composition of *Cannabis sativa* is constantly changing. New non-cannabinoid and cannabinoid constituents in the plant are discovered frequently. From 2005 to 2015, the number of cannabinoids identified in the whole plant increased from 70 to 104 and other known compounds in the plant increased from some 400 to around 650 (Izzo et al., 2009; ElSohly & Slade, 2005; Ahmed et al., 2008).

The cannabinoid that is primarily responsible for the psychoactive effects sought by cannabis users is THC (Gaoni & Mechoulam, 1964; Martin & Cone, 1999; Iversen, 2007). THC is found in a resin that covers the flowering tops and upper leaves of the female plant. Most of the other cannabinoids are either inactive or only weakly active, although some, such as CBD, may modify the psychoactive effects of THC (Mechoulam & Hanus, 2012).

The most common cannabis preparations are marijuana, hashish and hash oil. Marijuana is a herbal form of cannabis prepared from the dried flowering tops and leaves of the plant. Its potency depends on the growing conditions, the genetic characteristics of the plant, the ratio of THC to other cannabinoids, and the part of the plant that is used (Clarke & Watson, 2002). Cannabis plants may be grown to maximize their THC production by the "sinsemilla" method by which only female plants are grown together (Clarke & Watson, 2002).

Cannabis is typically smoked as marijuana in a hand-rolled cigarette or "joint", which may include tobacco to assist burning. A water pipe or "bong" is also a popular means of using all cannabis preparations (Hall & Degenhardt, 2009). Cannabis smokers typically inhale deeply and hold their breath to ensure maximum absorption of THC by the lungs.

One increasingly popular way of administrating cannabis is the use of vaporizers. Lower temperature vaporization of cannabis has been postulated as less harmful than smoking, as it may deliver fewer components of high molecular weight than smoked cannabis (Bloor et al., 2008). Whether vaporizing cannabis is a safer alternative to smoking remains uncertain, as the reduction in toxic smoke components needs to be weighed against the hazards of acute intoxication and long-term consequences to the brain (Wilsey et al., 2013; Eisenberg et al., 2014).

Inhalation by smoking or vaporization releases maximal levels of THC into the blood within minutes, peaking at 15–30 minutes and decreasing within 2–3 hours. Even with a fixed dose of THC in a cannabis cigarette, THC pharmacokinetics and effects vary as a function of the weight of the cannabis cigarette, the THC potency in the cigarette, its preparation, the concentration of other cannabinoids, the rate of inhalation, the depth and duration of puffs, the volume inhaled, the extent of breath-holding, the vital capacity and the escaped smoke and dose titration (Azorlosa, Greenwald & Stitzer, 1995; Azorlosa et al., 1992).

Hashish, once a general term for cannabis in the Eastern Mediterranean Region, now is being used to define cannabis resin (WHO, 1994). Hashish (derived from the resin of the flowering heads of the cannabis plant) may be mixed with tobacco and smoked as a joint or (typically in South Asia) it may be smoked in a clay pipe or *chillum* with or without tobacco, Hashish may also be cooked in foods and eaten. In India and other parts of South Asia, cannabis preparations from stalks and leaves, called *bhang*, is traditionally used as a drink or chewed and is part of religious and ritual use.

Survey data on patterns of cannabis use in most high- and middle-income countries indicates that most cannabis users smoke cannabis (Hall & Degenhardt, 2009). The chemistry and pharmacology of cannabis make it easiest to control doses when it is smoked (Iversen, 2007; Martin & Cone, 1999). Given the preponderance of smoking as the route of cannabis administration in developed countries, readers should assume throughout the remainder of this report that smoking is the method used unless otherwise stated.

2.1.3 Changes in cannabis potency

There has been an upward trend in the mean THC content of all confiscated cannabis preparations in the USA and in some European countries. The breeding of different strains has yielded plants and resins with dramatic increases in THC content over the past decade, from around 3% to 12–16% or higher (% of THC weight per dry weight of cannabis) with differences in different countries (Radwan et al., 2008; Niesink et al., 2015; Swift, et al., 2013; Zamengo, et al., 2014; Bruci, et al., 2012)

In the USA the THC content of cannabis increased from less than 2% in 1980 to 4.5% in 1997 and 8.5% in 2006 (ElSohly et al., 2000; ONDCP, 2007) to 8.8% in 2008 (Mehmedic et al., 2010). The increase in cannabis potency in the USA was mainly due to the increased potency of imported rather than domestically-produced cannabis (Mehmedic et al., 2010). In 2015, according to a number of USA laboratories, some retail cannabis seized by the US Drug Enforcement Administration (DEA) was found to contain 20% THC or more.

In 2011, cannabis resin at retail level in Europe was reported to have an average THC content that varied from 4% (Hungary) to 16% (Netherlands). According to the 2015 report of the European Monitoring Centre for Drugs and Drug Addiction (EMCDDA), 3–14% THC is the range of the THC content in herbal cannabis in Europe (2015a). Herbal cannabis produced by intensive indoor growing methods may have an average potency that is 2–3 times greater than that of imported herbal cannabis (EMCDDA, 2004). More recently in the European Union (EU), imported resin appears to be increasing in potency – possibly because resin producers are responding to the increased availability of high-potency domestically-produced herbal cannabis in the EU (EMCDDA, 2015b).

Hashish oil, a solvent-extracted liquid, is consumed by smoking, use of vaporization, or as a food additive. Users report more addictive behaviours and withdrawal symptoms with the high THC levels in hashish oil. In the USA hashish potencies did not increase consistently, with the mean annual potency varying from 2.5–9.2% in 1993–2003 to 12.0–29.3% in 2004–2008 (Mehmedic et al., 2010). Hashish oil potencies also varied considerably during this period, from a mean of 11.6 % in 1994 to a mean of 28.6% in 2000 to a mean of 19.4% the following year (Mehmedic et al., 2010).

2.1.4 Risk and protective factors

The terms "risk factors" and "protective factors" are widely used in public health. The term "risk factor" is used to describe individual or social factors that predict an increased risk of a disease or undesirable health condition. It is important to note that risk factors do not necessarily cause, but are associated with, the initiation of cannabis use, transitioning to frequent high-risk cannabis use and to the development of cannabis-use disorders.

Most of the studies on risk and protective factors for nonmedical use of cannabis and other drugs have been conducted in a small number of high-income countries such as Australia, Germany, Netherlands, New Zealand and the USA (Hawkins, Catalano &Miller, 1992; Stone et al., 2012; EMCDDA, 2015b). The limited studies in developing countries suggest that some of the same risk and protective factors also apply in these countries (Hall & Degenhardt, 2007). More research is needed to confirm that this is the case.

In developed countries the major social and contextual factors that increase the likelihood of initiation of cannabis use are drug availability, the use of tobacco and alcohol at an early age, and social norms that are tolerant of alcohol and drug use (Lascala, Friesthler & Gruenwald, 2005; Hawkins et al., 1992; Stone et al., 2012, EMCDDA, 2015). Overall, people from socially disadvantaged backgrounds are more likely to use illicit drugs (Daniel et al., 2009), although illicit drugs can also be commonly used in specific subgroups and party settings.

Family factors that are found to increase the risk of illicit drug use during adolescence include the poor quality of parent-child interaction and parent-child relationships, parental conflict, and parental and sibling drug use (Degenhardt et al., 2010; Fergusson, Boden & Horwood, 2015). However, there is no absolute relationship and not all adolescents growing up in families with these risk factors become illicit drug users.

Individual risk factors that increase the risk include: male gender (Ferguson, Horwood & Lynskey, 1994; Korhonen, et al., 2008); the personality traits of novelty (Cannon et al., 1993) and sensation seeking (Lipkus et al., 1994; Pinchevsky et al., 2012), peer early oppositional behaviour and conduct disorders in childhood (Lynskey, Fergusson & Horwood, 1994; Lynskey & Fergusson, 1995; Wymbs et al., 2012; Collins et al., 2011), poor school performance, low commitment to education and early school leaving (Townsend, Flisher & King, 2007; Lynskey & Hall, 2000; Tu, Ratner & Johnson, 2008) and inadequate sleep (Mednick, Christakis & Fowler, 2010). Associating with antisocial and drug-using peers is a strong predictor of adolescent alcohol and drug use (Fergusson, Boden & Horwood, 2008; Kandel & Andrews, 1987), independent of individual and family risk factors (Lynskey & Hall, 2000; Hawkins, Catalano & Miller, 1992). Figure 2.1 lists risk factors favourable to drug use.

In developed countries protective factors in childhood and adolescence are found to be positive family environments. Young adults who experienced strong parental support during adolescence are less likely to develop drug-use problems (King & Chassin, 2004; Stone et al., 2012). Perceptions of parental care play a key role in predicting cannabis use (Gerra et al., 2004). Good family management – encompassing effective monitoring, discipline, reward systems, reinforcement, etc. – is associated with lower rates of substance use among young adults (Stone et al., 2012). Religious involvement is associated with lower cannabis use and higher rates of abstinence in adolescents in most countries (Schulenberg et al., 2005). The same study (Schulenberg et al., 2005) also found that high scholastic achievement was associated with higher rates of abstinence from cannabis use.

Some factors are specifically associated with progression to dependence. These are found to be intensive or risky patterns of cannabis use, persistent use and early onset. Individuals who experienced positive effects of their early cannabis use (at age 14–16 years) had an increased risk of cannabis dependence later in life (Fergusson, Horwood & Beautrais, 2003). Also associated with the progression to dependence are various psychological and mental health factors (including low self-esteem, low self-control and low coping skills) and socioeconomic factors (including low socioeconomic status and a difficult financial situation) (Coffey et al., 2003; Fergusson, Horwood & Swain-Campbell, 2003; von Sydow et al., 2002).

Rates of cannabis dependence are higher among individuals reporting any lifetime psychiatric disorder, mood disorder, anxiety disorder, conduct disorder, personality disorder or attention deficit hyperactivity disorder (ADHD). Having a history of a substance use disorder (SUD) predicts development of an additional SUD. The transition to cannabis (or cocaine) dependence occurs considerably more quickly than the transition to nicotine or alcohol dependence (Lopez-Quintero et al., 2011).

Figure 2.1. Risk factors for drug use

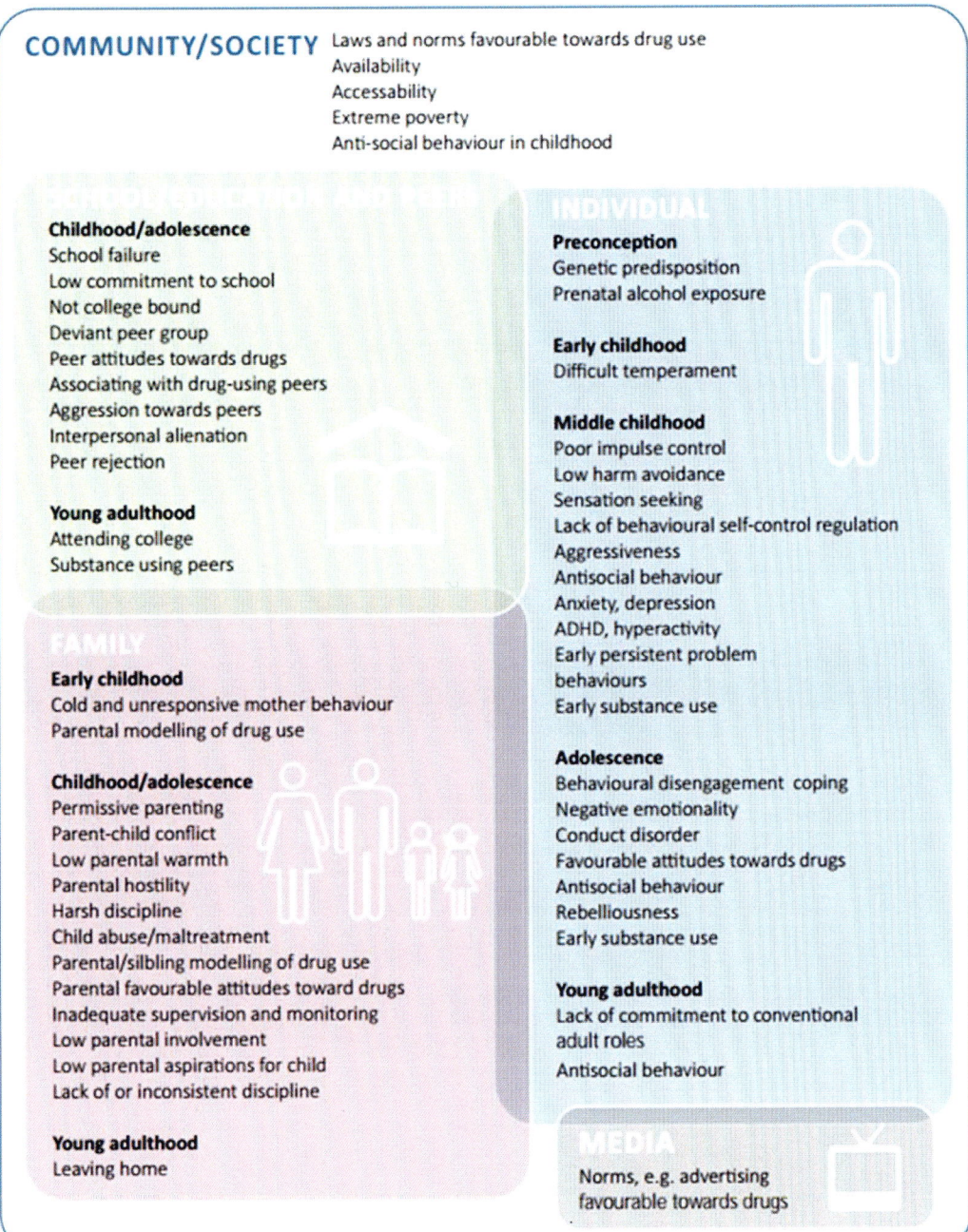

Source: UNODC, 2015, World Drug Report

2.1.5 Short-term health effects of cannabis use

The short-term effects of cannabis use are those that can occur shortly after a single occasion of use. These short-term effects depend on the dose received, the mode of administration, the user's prior experience with cannabis, any concurrent drug use, and the "set and setting" – i.e. the user's expectations, attitudes towards the effects of cannabis, mood state, and the social setting in which it is used (Fehr & Kalant, 1983).

In terms of short-term effects, it is implied that cannabis use precedes the effect, and that cannabis use and the effect occur closely together in time. When it is ethical to do so, these effects can be reproduced by administering cannabis under controlled conditions – for instance, in studies of the effects of cannabis use on cognitive performance and driving skills. These conditions apply to the short-term euphoric and relaxing effects sought by cannabis users and to some of its dysphoric effects (e.g. anxiety symptoms that are experienced by some users).

The most obvious short-term health effect of cannabis is intoxication marked by disturbances in the level of consciousness, cognition, perception, affect or behaviour, and other psychophysiological functions and responses. The magnitude of these effects will depend on the dose used, the route of administration, the setting and the mindset of the user (Brands et al., 1998). In this report, evidence is evaluated as to whether the short-term intoxicating effects of cannabis are possible causes of injuries, psychoses, suicidal behaviour and adverse physical health effects, such as stroke or acute coronary syndrome (See Box 2.1).

BOX 2.1. Acute cannabis intoxication

ICD–10 definition (WHO, 1993).

F12.0 Acute intoxication due to use of cannabinoids. A. The general criteria for acute intoxication (F1x.0) must be met.

B. There must be dysfunctional behaviour or perceptual abnormalities, including at least one of the following:

(1) euphoria and disinhibition;
(2) anxiety or agitation;
(3) suspiciousness or paranoid ideation;
(4) temporal showing (a sense that time is passing very slowly, and/or the person is experiencing a rapid flow of ideas;
(5) impaired judgement;
(6) impaired attention;
(7) impaired reaction time;
(8) auditory, visual, or tactile illusions;
(9) hallucinations with preserved orientation;
(10) depersonalization;
(11) derealization;
(12) interference with personal functioning.

C. At least one of the following signs must be present:

(1) increased appetite;
(2) dry mouth;
(3) conjunctival injection;
(4) tachycardia.

> **DSM-5 definition (APA, 2013)**
>
> Cannabis intoxication, a cannabis-related disorder coded as 292.89, is defined by DSM-5, as the following:
>
> - Recent use of cannabis
> - Clinically significant problematic behavioural or psychological changes (i.e. impaired motor coordination, euphoria, anxiety, sensation of slowed time, impaired judgment, social withdrawal) that developed during, or shortly after, cannabis use.
>
> At least 2 of the following signs, developing within 2 hours of cannabis use:
> - Conjunctival injection
> - Increased appetite
> - Dry mouth
> - Tachycardia
>   Symptoms not due to a general medical condition and not better accounted for by another mental disorder.

2.1.6 Long-term health effects of cannabis use

Long-term health effects are those that arise from regular cannabis use – especially daily use – over periods of months, years or decades. The time interval between the initiation of regular cannabis use and the development of long-term health effects may vary from several years to decades.

This report evaluates the evidence on whether long-term cannabis use is a contributory cause of the following health outcomes: dependence, cognitive impairment, mental disorders (psychoses, depression, anxiety and suicidal behaviour), and adverse physical health effects such as cardiovascular disease (CVD), chronic obstructive pulmonary disease and respiratory and other cancers. More information can be found in chapters 6 and 7 of this report.

2.1.7 Approach to making causal inferences

For this report, when judging the evidence on the adverse health effects of cannabis use, the criteria set out in Box 2.2 (Hall & Pacula, 2010) were used. The important contribution of Hill (1965) in his article *The environment and disease: association or causation?* is acknowledged.

The first criterion requires evidence of an association between cannabis use and the health outcome. This evidence can come from animal studies, human laboratory studies, case-control studies and prospective longitudinal epidemiological studies. As the consistency of the evidence of an association increases in various types of research studies, so does confidence in the existence of such an association.

The second requirement is evidence that makes reverse causation an implausible explanation of the association. We need to rule out the possibility that cannabis use is a consequence of the health outcome rather than a cause of it. The latter could be the case, for instance, if persons with clinical depression were more likely than non-depressed persons to use cannabis as a form of self-medication. This requirement can be satisfied by evidence from experiments (when they are ethically acceptable) and from prospective studies (when experiments are not ethically acceptable). Either type of study can show whether cannabis was used before the health outcome developed.

The third requirement is the most difficult to satisfy. This requires evidence that the association is not explained by other uncontrolled and unmeasured factors that increase the likelihood of persons both using cannabis and developing the health outcome that cannabis use is assumed to cause. This challenge arises because cannabis users (especially regular users) differ from non-users in various ways (apart from using cannabis) and these differences increase cannabis users' risks of experiencing adverse health and social outcomes independently of their cannabis use. Cannabis users are, for instance, more likely to use alcohol, tobacco and other illicit drugs than people who do not use cannabis (Kandel, 1993). They also differ from non-users in risk-taking, impulsivity, cognitive ability and other ways that increase their risk of adverse health outcomes such as accidents, using other illicit drugs or performing poorly in school (Fergusson, Boden & Horwood, 2015). These differences can make it difficult to be sure that adverse health outcomes that occur more often in regular cannabis users are caused by their cannabis use (Hall, 2015).

The most common method of addressing these inferential challenges has been by the statistical analysis of data from prospective studies to control for the effects of potentially confounding variables, such as other drug use and personal characteristics on which cannabis users differ from non-users (Hall, 2015). The major limitations of this approach are that not all studies have measured all plausible confounders and, when they have done so, these variables are measured with error, which prevents analyses from fully controlling for the effects of these variables. There may also be unmeasured factors that we do not know about and so do not measure in these studies (Costello & Angold, 2011; Richmond et al., 2014).

Mendelian randomization has been proposed as an approach to overcome this limitation of observational epidemiological studies (Davy Smith, 2011). This method uses genotypic information to approximate the design of a randomized control trial of the effects of the exposure via cannabis use (Richmond et al., 2014). This approach has not been applied to studying the health effects of cannabis because genetic studies have not yet identified common genotypes that are associated with cannabis use but not associated with the health outcomes under study (Kendler et al., 2012). The fourth requirement for making a causal inference is evidence that a causal relationship between cannabis use and the health outcome is biologically plausible (Hall & Pacula, 2010). This may come from animal or human experiments on the biological effects of cannabis use on brain and bodily functions and from detailed understandings of the neurobiology of the cannabinoid system and the pathophysiology of the health outcomes in question. Other factors that may support a causal interpretation include strength of the association, dose–response relationships, specificity of the association and reversibility of the effect after removal of the drug.

3. Epidemiology of cannabis use, disorders and treatment

3.1 What do we know?

3.1.1 Prevalence of cannabis use

3.1.1.1 Global and regional data

Cannabis is the most commonly used illicit drug globally (UNODC, 2015; WHO, 2010). The UNODC's World Drug Report 2015 shows the highest prevalence rates among Western Central Africa, North America, and Oceania (See Figure 3.1). The Global Burden of Disease study shows the highest age-standardized rates of use in Australasia and North America but a significant proportion of people using cannabis live in South and East Asia, followed by North America. Historically cannabis use and cultivation has been prevalent in Africa, Central Europe, South Asia and China from prehistoric times.

Figure 3.1. Annual prevalence of cannabis use for population aged 15–64 years

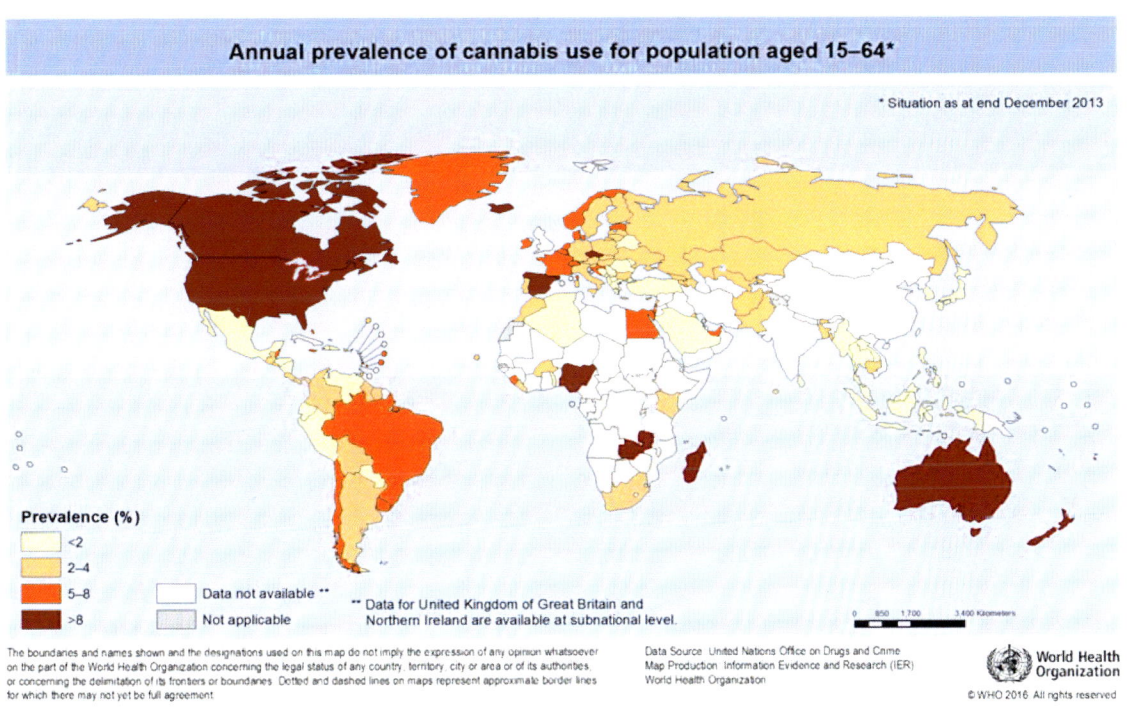

Source: World drug report 2015. United Nations Office on Drugs and Crime.

Today, there is still wide variation in the recorded prevalence of cannabis use within WHO regions. This in part reflects difficulties in collecting comparable data on illicit drug use. Some countries do not conduct surveys of drug use, some conduct surveys annually and others conduct them less frequently. Of those surveys that are conducted, there is variation between countries in assessing frequency of use, and age groups are divided differently or differ in the settings in which the adolescents and young adults are surveyed (e.g. schools vs. homes).

Nevertheless, there are some relatively good data on prevalence in some parts of the world. For instance, in the WHO European Region an estimated 14.6 million young Europeans (aged 15–34 years), or 11.7 % of this age group, used cannabis in the last year, with 8.8 million of these aged 15–24 years (15.2 % of this age group) (EMCDDA, 2015a). Levels of lifetime use differ considerably between countries, ranging from around one third of adults in Denmark, France and the United Kingdom, to 8% or less than 1 in 10 in Bulgaria, Romania and Turkey. Last-year use in this age group varied between 0.4 % and 22.1 %.

Herbal cannabis is becoming more popular in many EU countries – a trend driven by domestic production.

In the USA, the percentage of people aged 12 years or older who were current illicit drug users (8.4%) rose every year between 2002 and 2013 (SAMHSA, 2014). The higher percentage in 2014 than in prior years appears to reflect trends in cannabis use.

Measuring prevalence of cannabis use is difficult and it is even more difficult to measure how much cannabis, and the potency of that cannabis, is typically used by daily or less than daily users (Hall, 2015). There are no standard measures of the quantity used, and the average THC content of cannabis in most countries and regions is unknown. Epidemiological studies have used daily or near-daily cannabis use as an approximate measure of heavy use.

In high-income countries, such as the USA, cannabis use usually begins in the mid-to-late teens. Heaviest use occurs in the early twenties and declines throughout the late twenties into the early thirties. About 10% of people who use cannabis become daily users and another 20–30% use it weekly.

3.1.1.2 Country examples

Most data on the patterns and health consequences of cannabis use has been collected in high-income countries in Europe, North America and Oceania. The earliest systematic study of cannabis use was the Indian Hemp Commission in 1894 and the earliest descriptions of cannabis-induced psychosis were by Chopra (Chopra, Chopra & Chopra, 1942). At the WHO expert meeting on cannabis in Stockholm in April 2015, various experts presented national and regional prevalence data. The following examples are from those countries that have data on prevalence and patterns of cannabis use that were presented at the Stockholm meeting.

Brazil

The prevalence of use in the last 12 months in Brazil is 2.5% in the adult population and 3.5% in the adolescent population, a rate similar to that in other Latin American countries (UNIAD/INPAD, 2012). Lifetime use was 4.3% among adolescents and 6.8% among adults (UNIAD/INPAD, 2012). The national school survey found that 7.3% of students reported illicit drug use at least once in their lifetime (Horta et al., 2014). The highest rates of cannabis use are in young single males, adults who are unemployed, adults with a higher income, and individuals living in large cities (Jungerman et al., 2009).

Chile and neighbouring countries

Chile has one of the highest rates of cannabis use in Latin America. Until recently Chile's prevalence was lower than Uruguay's and never exceeded 6 % of the general population in past-year use. Past-year use in the general population has increased to 11.3% (SENDA, 2015). Since 2011, the prevalence of use has increased significantly in Chile, with 30.6% of students in school surveys reporting use in the past year (Castillo-Carniglia 2014, SENDA, 2014). A similar trend has occurred in Uruguay, where cannabis use in the general population grew from 1.4% to 8.3% over 10 years. In contrast, Peru has the lowest prevalence of past year use in the region at around 1% (CICAD/OEA, 2015).

In Chile and other Latin American countries, the herbal form of cannabis is the most usual form, but a third of the Chilean cannabis market is "pressed marijuana". This is a dried form of cannabis leaves, pressed with varying unidentified components such as glue, honey and tobacco, that comes mainly from Paraguay (SENDA, 2013).

Kenya

Cannabis is referred to in Kenya as *bhang* and is prepared from the leaves and stems of the cannabis plant. It is commonly smoked in powder form or consumed as a beverage. It grows easily in the Mt. Kenya area and is readily available (NACADA, 2007). The NACADA rapid assessment of substance abuse in Kenya (2012) found that *bhang* was more common among urban residents, the unemployed and among men. Use has decreased since 2007 in the general population (6.5% ever use in 2007 reduced to 5.4% ever use in 2012) but has increased among 10–14-year-olds (from 0.3% in 2007 to 1.1% in 2012). Although urban youth and adults are more likely to use *bhang*, rural use has been on the rise (NACADA, 2012). Within the 15–24-year-old age category, 1.5% of individuals are currently using *bhang*. As in higher-income countries, cannabis use in Kenya is most common among 18–25-year-olds and falls dramatically in the mid-thirties (NACADA, 2012).

Morocco

Household surveys conducted in Morocco in 2004–2005 found a past-month prevalence for cannabis use of 4% (Kadri et al., 2010). In 2013, the results of MEDSPAD (the Mediterranean School Survey Project on Alcohol and Other Drugs) showed that, among 15–17-year-old secondary school students, lifetime use of cannabis was 9.5% for boys and 2.1% for girls, and past-month use was 5.8% for boys and 0.6% for girls. Cannabis use increased with age and was consistently higher among males than females. The mean age of onset in the 2013 MEDSPAD sample was 14.9 years (El Omari & Toufiq, 2015).

South Africa

The National Survey of Youth Risk Behaviour indicates that 12.8% of South African students in grades 8–10 (13–15-year-olds) have used cannabis, and 9.2% did so in the past month (Bhana, 2015). A study of young people in grades 8–10 in the Western Cape in South Africa found lifetime use of 23.6%. The South African Stress and Health Study (SASH) surveyed over 4000 adults aged 18 years and up in a household survey and found 8.4% lifetime use. In all studies summarized by Bhana (2015), males were more likely to use than females, and urban dwellers more likely to use than their non-urban counterparts.

3.1.2 Prevalence of cannabis-use disorders

Harmful use of cannabis and dependence are the most common drug-use disorders in epidemiological surveys in Australia, Canada and the USA. Cannabis-use disorder is estimated to affect 1–2% of adults in the past year and 4–8% of adults during their lifetime (Hall & Pacula, 2010; Anthony, 2006). The risk of developing dependence among those who have ever used cannabis was estimated at 9% in the USA in the early 1990s (Anthony, 2006) compared to 32% for nicotine, 23% for heroin, 17% for cocaine, 15% for alcohol and 11% for stimulants (Anthony, Warner & Kessler, 1994).

Approximately 13.1 million people are cannabis-dependent globally (Degenhardt et al., 2013). Global prevalence of cannabis dependence in the general population is below half a percent but there is considerable variation, with higher prevalence in high-income countries where some of the more recent studies showed higher rates of 1–2% (NIH, 2015).

According to the Global Burden of Disease study (Degenhardt et al., 2013); males have higher cannabis dependence prevalence rates (0.23% [0.20–0.27%]) than females (0.14% [0.12–0.16%]), Women exhibit an accelerated progression to cannabis-use disorder after first use, and show more adverse clinical problems than men do (Cooper & Haney, 2014). Prevalence peaks in the 20–24 years age group at between 0.4% and 3.4% among males, and between 0.2% and 1.9% among females in all regions. It thereafter decreases steadily with age. There are some indications that prevalence of cannabis dependence increased worldwide between 2001 and 2010 (Degenhardt et al., 2013).

The USA is one of few countries to have collected epidemiological data on prevalence of cannabis-use disorders in a consistent manner over time. The prevalence of cannabis-use disorders increased in the USA between 1991–1992 and 2001–2002 (Compton et al., 2004) while the prevalence of cannabis use remained stable. The prevalence of cannabis use more than doubled between 2001–2002 and 2012–2013, and there was a large increase in the prevalence of cannabis-use disorders during that time. The past-year prevalence of DSM-IV cannabis use disorder was 1.5% (0.08) in 2001–2002 and 2.9% (SE, 0.13) in 2012–2013 ($P < .05$). While not all cannabis users experience problems, nearly 3 out of 10 cannabis users manifested a cannabis-use disorder in 2012–2013. Because the risk for cannabis-use disorders did not increase among users, the increase in prevalence of cannabis-use disorders is due to an increase in prevalence of users in the adult population of the USA. With few exceptions, increases in the prevalence of cannabis-use disorders between 2001–2002 and 2012–2013 were also statistically significant ($P < .05$) across demographic subgroups. (Hasin et al., 2015).

Pooled estimates suggest that the remission rate for cannabis dependence is 17% per annum (Calabria et al., 2010).

3.1.3 Treatment trends

According to WHO data, 16% of countries included in the recent ATLAS survey (Atlas 2015 in press) reported cannabis use as the main reason for people seeking substance abuse treatment. This puts cannabis second only to alcohol as a reason for treatment entry.

The number of persons seeking treatment for cannabis-use disorders and associated conditions have increased since the 1990s in many developed and some developing countries. Cannabis is now the drug of primary concern in a significant proportion of treatment episodes in the UNODC regions of Africa, Oceania, the USA and EU (UNODC, 2015). The number of cannabis users seeking help has increased over the past two decades in Australia, Europe and the USA (EMCDDA, 2015a; Roxburgh et al., 2010; WHO, 2010).

The widespread use of cannabis across the EU and the increase in the use of the drug in recent years is reflected in the high number of cannabis users now seeking treatment in Europe (Figure 3.2). In 2012, 110 000 of those enrolling in specialized drug treatment in the EU reported cannabis as the primary drug for which treatment was being sought. Cannabis is the second most commonly reported primary drug in both inpatient (18% of clients) and outpatient (26% of clients) treatment settings (EMCDDA, 2015b). For instance, in 2011 cannabis was the primary drug problem of 48% of persons entering drug treatment, and of 58% of new treatment entrants in the Netherlands (EMCDDA, 2014). It is uncertain how much increased treatment-seeking may be linked to the use of higher-THC cannabis products in, for instance, the Netherlands and the USA (Hall, 2015).

Figure 3.2. New clients entering treatment by primary drugs, 2006–2013

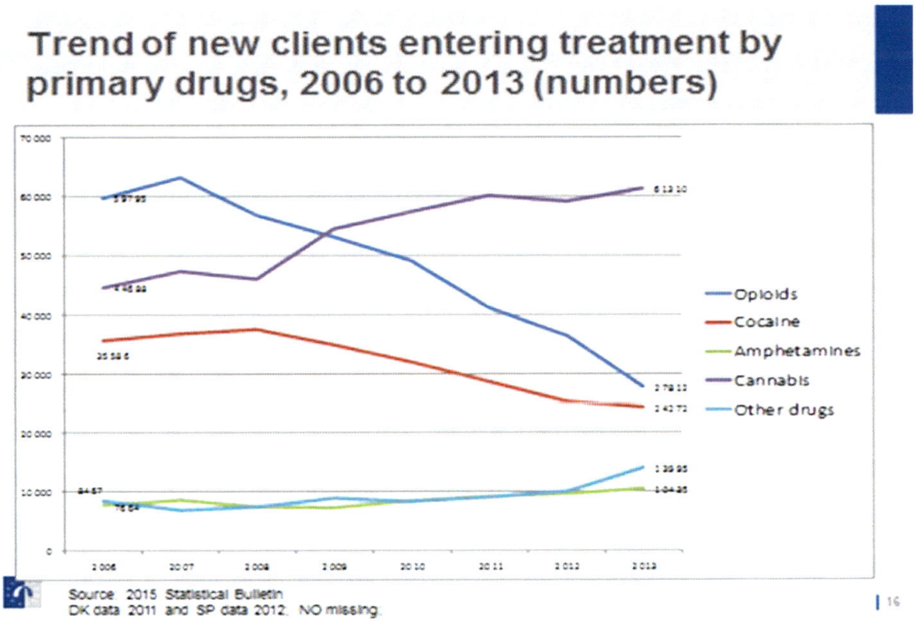

Source: EMCDDA (2015c). Statistical bulletin. Lisbon: European Monitoring Centre for Drugs and Drug Addiction (http://www.emcdda.europa.eu/data/stats2015, accessed 16 February 2016.)

Emergency departments reported that, from 2004 to 2011, for cannabis alone or in combination with other drugs, cannabis involvement in managed cases increased substantially. Cannabis thus represents 36% of all illicit drug use that is mentioned in the

USA and 31% mentioned in an urban emergency department in Switzerland (SAMHSA, 2011; Liakoni et al., 2015). In a consortium of 16 sentinel centres across Europe reporting acute drug toxicity presentations in emergency departments, cannabis ranked third among drugs after heroin and cocaine (Dines et al., 2015b). It has also been reported that cannabis is a small but increasing burden on emergency services in Australia (Kaar et al., 2015). There are indications from the USA and the EU that acute cannabis-induced physical symptoms, anxiety and sometimes psychotic symptoms are among the reasons that illicit drug users present to hospital emergency departments (Dines et al., 2015a; Liakoni et al., 2015; SAMHSA, 2009; Davis et al., 2015).

In some countries treatment uptake is also likely to have been influenced by an increased availability and diversity of treatment options for cannabis users, as well as greater recognition among service providers of the need to address problems related to the consumption of this drug.

There have also been some changes in the age structure of persons seeking treatment by primary drug. Figures 3.3 and 3.4, which are based on data from 26 European countries, show the age structure of clients entering treatment by primary drug in 2006 and 2013.

Figure 3.3. Age structure of clients entering treatment by primary drug, 2006

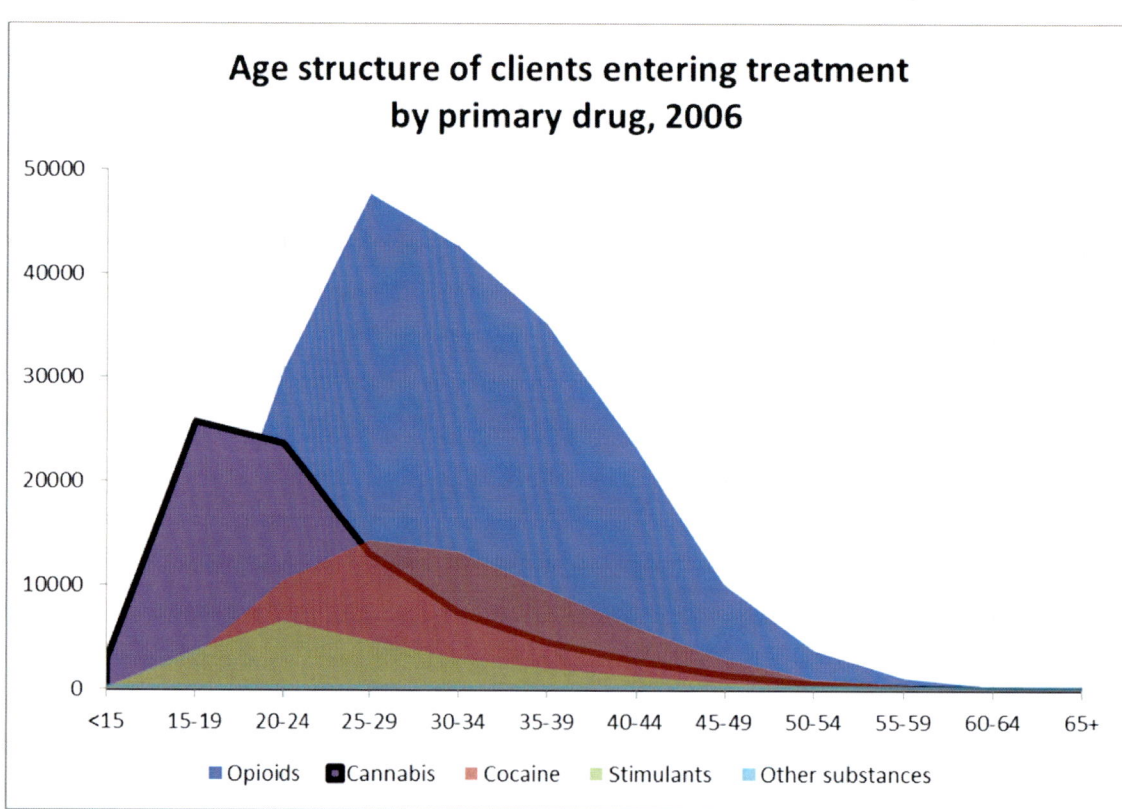

Figure 3.4. Age structure of clients entering treatment by primary drug, 2013

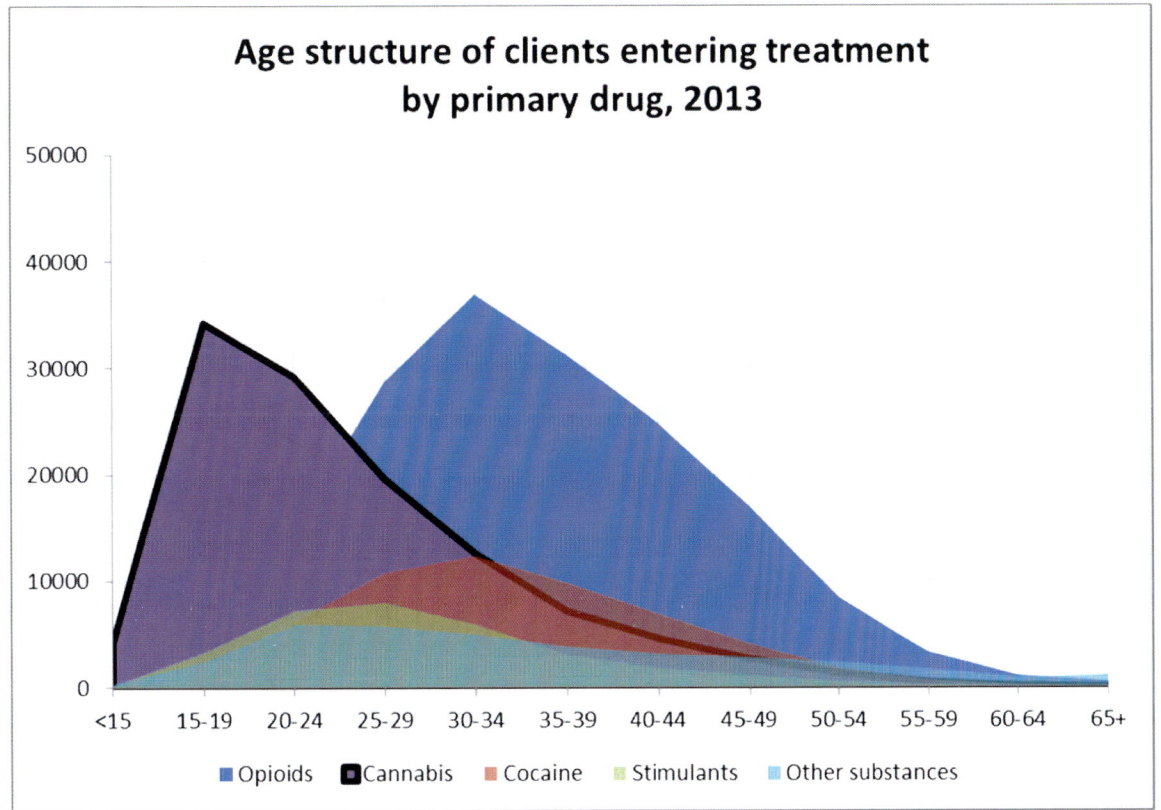

Source: EMCDDA (2015a), European drug report 2015; and EMCDDA (2015c), Statistical bulletin. Lisbon: European Monitoring Centre for Drugs and Drug Addiction (available at http://www.emcdda.europa.eu/data/stats2015, accessed 16 February 2016).

The adverse health and social consequences of cannabis use reported by cannabis users who seek treatment for dependence appear to be less severe than those reported by persons dependent on alcohol or opioid (Hall & Pacula, 2010; Degenhardt & Hall, 2012). However, rates of recovery from cannabis dependence among those seeking treatment are similar to those treated for alcohol dependence (Florez-Salamanca et al., 2013).

3.1.4 Areas that require more research

- Global data are required on the frequency of cannabis use (more than once daily, daily, near daily, weekly, etc.) and the prevalence of health and social consequences.
- Data are also required on the typical doses of THC and other cannabinoids (e.g. cannabidiol or CBD) that users receive through different modes of use (smoked, vaporized, ingested). There are limited data on cannabis potency trends over time and their impact on health (e.g. cognition, psychosis, accidents, motivation, emergency department mentions, cannabis-use disorders).

- Most epidemiological research on cannabis has focused on smokers in a small number of high-income countries. More research is needed on cannabis use in low- and middle-income countries.
- Global assessments are needed of the relationship between cannabis use and the use of other drugs.
- Cannabis and tobacco are often mixed together and there is a need for more data from well-designed studies on the prevalence and health consequences of :
    - smoked cannabis only;
    - different routes of cannabis administration;
    - potential added health risks from the use of cannabis in combination with tobacco;
    - the THC and other cannabis preparations, including pressed marijuana, in different parts of the world (e.g. in Latin American countries, and at different periods of time).
- Most of the studies on risk and protective factors for cannabis use have been conducted in a limited number of high-income countries. There is some uncertainty as to whether the same risk factors apply in low- and middle-income countries.
- Global data are lacking on trends in the prevalence of harmful cannabis use and of cannabis dependence (cannabis-use disorders).

4. Neurobiology of cannabis use

4.1 What do we know?

4.1.1 The psychoactive components and neurobiology of cannabis use

The principal psychoactive component of *Cannabis sativa,* THC (Iversen, 2012), acts on specific receptors in the brain. These receptors also respond to naturally-occurring cannabinoids (known as endogenous cannabinoids or endocannabinoids) such as anandamide (Iversen, 2012). The endocannabinoids regulate the actions of neurotransmitters that play roles in human and animal cognition, emotion and memory (Cascio & Pertwee, 2012).

Two types of cannabinoid receptors have been identified on which THC acts: type 1 (CB_1) and type 2 (CB_2) cannabinoid receptors. CB_1 receptors are found primarily in the brain where they are most concentrated in regions involved in memory (hippocampus), emotional responses (amygdala), cognition (cerebral cortex), motivation (the limbic forebrain) and motor coordination (cerebellum) (Hu & Mackie, 2015; Iversen, 2012). CB_2 receptors are found primarily in the body where they seem to play a role in the regulation of the immune system (Iversen, 2012) and have multiple other functions, including acting on the gastrointestinal tract, liver, heart, muscle, skin and reproductive organs (Madras, 2015). The CB_1 receptors play a key role in the psychoactive effects of cannabis. Drugs that block the actions of CB_1 receptors block the cannabis high in humans and stop animals from self-administering cannabis (Huestis et al., 2001; Iversen, 2012).

The brain's dopamine reward pathway contains both CB_1 and CB_2 receptors. Animal and human studies indicate that these receptors respond to THC by increasing dopamine release, an effect that probably explains the euphoric effects of cannabis. THC produces a smaller dopamine release than cocaine or methamphetamines, but dopamine release happens more quickly with cannabis because cannabis is typically smoked (Volkow, 2015). THC can be detected in plasma within seconds of smoking cannabis and it has a half-life of two hours. Peak plasma levels of THC are around 100 μg/L after smoking 10-15 mg of cannabis over a 5-7 minute period. THC is highly lipophilic and is distributed throughout the body (Moffat AC, Osselton MD, Widdop B, 2004).

Dopamine is involved in the control of cognition, attention, emotionality and motivation (Bloomfield et al., 2014). Cannabis alters time perception and coordination by acting on cannabinoid receptors in the basal ganglia, frontal cortex and cerebellum, which are brain regions involved in motor control and memory. Cannabis also affects psychomotor function. It impairs movement and coordination, manipulation and dexterity, grace, strength and speed. Evidence suggests that recent smoking and/or blood THC concentrations 2–5 ng/mL are associated with substantial driving impairment, particularly in occasional smokers (Hartman & Huestis, 2013) The effects of cannabis on the cerebellum probably explain the driving impairment produced by cannabis (Volkow et al., 2014a), which is described in detail in section 5.1. Animal and human studies show that cognitive and psychomotor functions are impaired directly after cannabis use (Iversen, 2012) and these impairments can persist for several days after use (Crean, Crane & Mason, 2011; Volkow et al., 2014a).

4.1.2 Neurobiology of long-term cannabis use

The daily use of cannabis over years and decades appears to produce persistent impairments in memory and cognition, especially when cannabis use begins in adolescence (Meier et al., 2012; Volkow et al., 2014a). The neurobiology of the cannabinoid system suggests that these effects may arise because chronic THC use reduces the number of CB_1 receptors (i.e. "down-regulates" these receptors) in brain regions that are involved in memory and cognition (Iversen, 2012) Experimental studies suggest that animals exposed to THC during puberty may be more susceptible to these effects of cannabis (Schneider, 2012).

Brain imaging studies comparing school students who are regular long-term cannabis users and non-using students typically find poorer cognitive performance and large decreases in perfusion in the former using SPECT scans (Mena et al., 2013). These changes could partially explain the lower educational attainment and lower grades among chronic cannabis users (Volkow et al., 2014a) and are discussed in more detail in section 6.1.2.

Magnetic resonance imaging (MRI) studies have found structural differences between the brains of chronic adult cannabis users and the brains of non-using controls. Changes can be seen in the grey/white matter, in global brain measures (Batalla et al., 2013), and in connectivity (Lopez-Larson, Rogowska & Yurgelun-Todd, 2015). Structural brain abnormalities are seen in CB_1-rich areas involved in cognitive functions. In addition, reduced hippocampal volume has been found in neuroimaging studies (Ashtari et al., 2011; Cousijn et al., 2012; Matochik et al., 2005; Yücel et al., 2008). In some studies these reductions persist after abstinence (Ashtari et al., 2011) and have been associated with impaired memory

(Lorenzetti et al., 2015). Neuroimaging studies have also found reduced volumes in the amygdala, the cerebellum and frontal cortex in chronic cannabis users (Batalla et al., 2013; Yücel et al., 2008). In a large study population (1574 participants), in which cortical thickness was measured by MRI, an association was found between cannabis use in early adolescence and reduced cortical thickness in male participants with a high polygenic risk score. Adults who have smoked cannabis since adolescence show reduced neuronal connectivity in the prefrontal areas responsible for executive functioning and inhibitory control and in the subcortical networks that are responsible for habits and routines (Volkow et al., 2014a). The precuneous – a node involved in integration of various brain functions such as awareness and alertness – is particularly affected in frequent cannabis users. Long-term cannabis use is hazardous to the white matter of the developing brain, with evidence of axon connectivity damage in three fibre tracts: the hippocampus (right fimbria), the splenium of the corpus callosum, and commissural fibres (which connect the two halves of the cerebral hemispheres). Damage was higher with younger age of onset of regular cannabis use (Volkow et al., 2014a).

The fimbria is a part of the hippocampus involved in learning and memory (Zalesky et al., 2012). These findings are consistent with the observation that impaired memory is a common complaint among cannabis users seeking treatment (Hall, 2015). Recovery of hippocampal connectivity after long-term abstinence has been reported (Yücel et al., 2016). Atypical orbitofrontal functional connectivity patterns were observed in attentional/executive, motor and reward networks in adolescents with heavy cannabis use. These anomalies may be reflected in suboptimal decision-making capacity and increased impulsivity (Lopez-Larson, Rogowska & Yurgelun-Todd, 2015). Chronic cannabis use has also been shown to reduce the brain's capacity to synthesize or release dopamine (Bloomfield et al., 2014), which could explain why cannabis users have higher scores on negative emotionality (Volkow et al., 2014b).

4.1.3 Neurobiology of prenatal cannabis exposure

Polydrug use makes it difficult to study the effects of cannabis on child development since the effects of other drugs, both illicit and legal, may influence study outcomes. A large multicentre study with over 10 000 pregnant women participating found that polydrug use was common among women who use drugs. Specifically, they found that 93% of all women who used, for instance, cocaine or opiates during pregnancy also used alcohol, tobacco and/or cannabis (Konijnenberg, 2015).

Nevertheless, accumulating evidence suggests that prenatal cannabis exposure may interfere with normal development and maturation of the brain. Children exposed to cannabis in utero demonstrate impaired attention, learning and memory, impulsivity and behavioural problems and a higher likelihood of using cannabis when they mature (Sonon et al., 2015; Noland et al., 2005; Goldschmidt, Day & Richardson, 2000; Goldschmidt et al., 2004; Goldschmidt et al., 2008; Day, Leech & Goldschmidt, 2011).

In animal studies, prenatal exposure to THC shows that it can make the brain's reward system more sensitive to the effects of other drugs (DiNieri & Hurd, 2012). Human research has suggested that cannabis exposure in utero may alter regulation of the mesolimbic dopamine system in children (DiNieri et al., 2011). Children exposed to cannabis prenatally also have higher rates of neurobehavioural and cognitive impairments (Tortoriello, 2014) that may be related to the impaired formation of axonal connections between neurons during fetal development (Volkow, 2014a). Importantly, the negative effects of prenatal drug exposure may not become apparent until later in development. It is, therefore, essential to follow up cannabis-exposed children long into adolescence, and human research in this domain is still limited, which contrasts with nicotine or alcohol research.

4.1.4 Neurobiology of cannabis effects in adolescence

Accumulating evidence reveals that regular, heavy cannabis use during adolescence is associated with more severe and persistent negative outcomes than use during adulthood. As mentioned in section 3.1.2, the risk of dependence has been estimated at 16% in those who initiated cannabis use in adolescence (Anthony, 2006) and 33–50% in daily cannabis users (van der Pol et al., 2013).

The adolescent brain seems to be more vulnerable to cannabis than the adult brain, and early initiation of heavy use appears to disrupt the trajectory of normal brain development. Heavy or regular adolescent cannabis users manifest a range of cognitive deficits, including impairments in attention, learning and memory, and an inability to switch ideas or responses. These deficits are similar in adults, but in adolescents they are more likely to persist and may recover only after longer periods of abstinence (Fried, Watkinson & Gray, 2005). Earlier onset users show greater impairment in cognitive domains, including learning and memory, attention and other executive functions (Pope et al., 2003; Gruber et al., 2012). Decrements in cognitive function are correlated with initiation of cannabis use during adolescence (Pope et al., 2003).

A recent large-scale longitudinal study followed a large cohort from childhood to 38 years of age and assessed neuropsychological functioning at multiple time points. The study revealed that adolescents who used cannabis weekly, or harboured a cannabis-use disorder before the age of 18, showed larger neuropsychological decline and I.Q. reduction than those who became dependent during adulthood (Meier et al., 2012). The results are consistent with cross-sectional findings in adult populations, and reinforce the conclusion that sustained abstinence may not enable cognitive functional recovery if use was initiated during adolescence. A subsequent re-analysis showed that socioeconomic differences did not account for the sustained loss of I.Q. (Moffitt et al., 2013; Solowij et al., 2011).

As noted in section 4.1.1, the CB_1 and CB_2 receptors are expressed in the brain and peripheral tissues (Mackie, 2005). In the brain, CB_1 receptors are the most abundant of the G-protein coupled receptors and mediate most, if not all, of the psychoactive effects of THC in cannabis. CB_2 receptors in the brain also modulate the release of chemical signals primarily engaged in immune system functions (e.g. cytokines). Brain imaging has generally revealed changes in the brains of adolescents or adults who initiated cannabis use during adolescence (Lorenzetti et al., 2013; Bossong et al., 2014; Jacobus & Tapert, 2014). Frequent cannabis use is associated with smaller whole brain and hippocampus size, reduced cortical grey matter, and insular cortical thickness that varies in accordance with level of use (Churchwell, Lopez-Larson & Yurgelun-Todd, 2010; Lopez-Larson et al., 2011). Some studies found correlations between brain changes and deficits in learning and memory (Ashtari et al., 2011). Age of onset of cannabis use is apparently not as important in causing hippocampal shrinkage as the amount or frequency of use (Lorenzetti et al., 2014). Changes in cortical volume may predate and predispose individuals to use cannabis, but this is unlikely for changes in the hippocampus (Cheetham et al., 2012) which seems vulnerable to heavy cannabis use, regardless of age.

Studies in rodents have shown that long-term exposure to cannabinoids during adolescence decreases dopamine release in the brain's reward regions (Pistis et al., 2004; Schneider, 2012). The effects of early cannabis use on dopamine pathways could possibly, in addition to environmental risk factors, explain the role of cannabis as an apparent "gateway drug" – i.e. a drug whose early use increases the risk of later use of other illicit drugs (see also section 6.1.3.2). Early alcohol and nicotine use can also function as gateways for cannabis use by priming the brain to produce elevated dopamine responses to cannabis and other drugs, though alternative explanations based on the overall susceptibility to drug-taking behaviour and higher accessibility of marijuana cannot be excluded (Volkow, 2014b).

4.1.5 Modifiers of risk: the interplay between genetics and environment

The acute and long-term effects of cannabis use depend on interactions between genetic predispositions and environmental factors (Danielsson et al., 2015). Individuals with certain personality profiles may be more likely to use cannabis – particularly those who score higher on sensation-seeking (Muro & Rodríguez, 2015), extraversion and neuroticism, or on adolescent aggression scales, and those who engage in antisocial behaviour (Hayatbakhsh et al., 2009). See also section 2.1.4 on risk and protective factors.

A meta-analysis of twin studies estimated that, among males, 51% of problematic cannabis use could be attributed to shared genes, 20% to a shared environment and 29% to an unshared environment. Among females, 59% was attributed to genetics, 15% to a shared environment, and 26% to an unshared environment (Verweij et al., 2010).

A gene variant of cannabinoid receptor 1 (CNR1) has been associated with cannabis-related problems among frequent users. This variant appears to moderate the relationship between trait impulsivity and cannabis-related problems. Individuals who frequently use cannabis and who have the CNR1 risk variants have higher trait impulsivity and have a higher risk of developing problems related to their cannabis use (Bidwell et al., 2013).

Gerra and colleagues found that serotonin transporter (5-HTT) gene variants were related to cannabis initiation but the environment played a larger role via the stressful effects of perceived parental neglect, a factor consistently related to initiation of cannabis use (Gerra et al., 2010). Lack of parental control and support increases the probability of cannabis initiation by interacting with emotional stability and extraversion (Creemers et al., 2015).

4.1.6 Areas that require more research

Much of the research on the neurobiological effects of cannabis involves persons who are either still heavy cannabis users or who have only recently stopped using cannabis. This makes it difficult to know if the neurobiological effects, and specifically the cognitive impairments, found in these users improve after a year or more of abstinence. The available limited evidence is mixed. Some studies have found persistent impairments while others have found that impairments improve significantly with prolonged abstinence (Solowij & Pesa, 2012; Meier M et al., 2012).

- Better studies are needed to assess the degree of cognitive recovery in regular cannabis users after sustained abstinence, as a function of age of onset of use, THC potency, frequency of use and similar parameters.
- "Reverse translational" research is needed to verify, in animals, whether observed changes in human brain structure or function (e.g. dopamine release) can be replicated using cannabis or THC.
- Both human and animal studies require confirmation by multiple groups using sufficiently large numbers of subjects to yield robust statistical significance. In research on the effects of prenatal cannabis exposure, it is essential to follow up cannabis-exposed children long into adolescence.
- There is need for large-scale longitudinal research on adolescents, beginning prior to drug initiation and continuing long into adulthood.

5. Short-term effects of cannabis

5.1 What do we know?

5.1.1 Cognition and coordination

Crean, Crane & Mason (2011) reviewed a broad spectrum of cognitive functions, designated as executive functions, and identified studies that reported that attention, concentration, decision-making, impulsivity, inhibition (self-control of responses), reaction time, risk taking, verbal fluency and working memory were impaired acutely in a dose-dependent manner, although these effects were not consistently observed.

Cannabis acutely impairs several components of cognitive function, with the most robust effects on short-term episodic and working memory, planning and decision-making, response speed, accuracy and latency (Ranganathan & D'Souza, 2006). Some studies also report increased risk-taking and impulsivity (Crean, Crane & Mason, 2011). Less experienced cannabis users undergo stronger intoxicating effects on attention and concentration than those with established drug tolerance. Cannabis also acutely impairs motor coordination, interferes with driving skills and increases the risk of injuries. Evidence suggests that recent cannabis smoking is associated with substantial driving impairment, particularly in occasional smokers, with implications for work in safety-sensitive positions or when operating a means of transportation, including aircraft (Hartman & Huestis, 2013). Complex human/machine performance can be impaired as long as 24 hours after smoking a moderate dose of cannabis and the user may be unaware of the drug's influence (Leirer, Yesavage & Morrow, 1991).

5.1.2 Anxiety and psychotic symptoms

A minority of first-time cannabis users become very anxious have panic attacks, experience hallucinations and vomit. These symptoms may be sufficiently distressing to prompt affected users to seek medical care (Smith, 1968; Thomas, 1993; Weil, 1970). Experienced users may also have negative experiences if they use more potent cannabis products than usual, or use cannabis by an unfamiliar route (e.g. oral ingestion) that does not permit them to achieve their usual dose of THC. Hallucinations may occur after using very high doses of THC, and may occur at lower doses in individuals with a pre-existing vulnerability to psychosis (e.g. having experienced psychotic symptoms or having a first-degree relative with a psychotic disorder). These distressing experiences are often time-limited and can usually be managed by reassurance and mild sedation in a safe environment (Dines et al., 2015).

5.1.3 Acute toxicity

The risk of a fatal cannabis overdose is extremely small compared to the risks of opioid and stimulant drug overdoses (Gable, 2004). The dose of THC that reliably kills rodents is extremely high and the equivalent fatal dose in humans extrapolated from animal studies is between 15 g (Gable, 2004) and 70 g (Iversen, 2007; Lachenmeier & Rehm, 2015). This is much greater than the amount of cannabis that a very heavy user would consume in a day (Gable, 2004). There are no reports of fatal overdoses in the epidemiological literature (Calabria et al., 2010b). The lack of respiratory overdoses is consistent with the absence of cannabinoid receptors in brain stem areas that control respiration (Iversen, 2012).

5.1.4 Acute cardiovascular effects

Acute exposure to cannabis increases heart rate and blood pressure and can in some cases cause orthostatic hypotension (Pacher & Kunos, 2013; Schmid et al., 2010). There have been case reports of serious cardiovascular complications, including acute coronary syndromes and strokes, in cannabis users (Jouanjus, 2014). Mittleman and colleagues found that the risk of myocardial infarction was four times higher in patients with a recent myocardial infarction in the hour after smoking cannabis compared to cannabis users without a history of myocardial infarction (Mittleman et al., 2001). The risk then declined rapidly. Many of these more serious events have been reported in heavy daily cannabis smokers and are discussed in more detail in section 7.1.2.

5.1.5 Acute effects on lungs and airways

The acute bronchial effects of smoking tobacco and smoking cannabis differ; tobacco smoking produces acute bronchial constriction, while cannabis smoking causes acute bronchial dilation in proportion to the dose of THC (Tashkin, 2015).This effect has been reported in cannabis users in the United States where cannabis used to be smoked alone Users in many parts of the world frequently smoke cannabis and tobacco together (especially when cannabis resin is used), and this combination is likely to produce different acute bronchial effects. The effects of long-term cannabis smoking on lung function are considered in more detail in section 7.1.1.

5.1.6 Traffic injuries and fatalities

At the time of the last WHO report on cannabis (WHO, 1997), laboratory studies showed that cannabis and THC produced dose-related impairments in reaction time, information processing, perceptual-motor coordination, motor performance, attention and tracking behaviour (Moskowitz, 1985; Robbe & O'Hanlon, 1993). These findings suggested that cannabis could potentially cause car crashes if users drove while intoxicated.

It was unclear in 1997, however, if cannabis use increased traffic accidents. Studies in driving simulators indicated that cannabis-impaired drivers were aware of their impairment and compensated by slowing down and taking fewer risks. There were similar findings in the small number of studies on the effects of cannabis use on driving on the road (Smiley, 1999). In some of these studies, however, cannabis-impaired drivers responded less effectively to simulated emergencies than control drivers did (Robbe, 1994).

Most epidemiological studies of traffic fatalities in the 1990s are reported only on the presence of cannabis metabolites. These indicated only that cannabis had been used hours to days before the accident; they did not establish that the drivers were impaired by cannabis at the time of the accident. Moreover, a substantial proportion of drivers with cannabis in their blood also had high blood alcohol concentrations (BACs), which made it difficult to distinguish the effects of cannabis and alcohol on accident risk (Hall, Solowij & Lemon, 1994).

In the past two decades, better designed epidemiological studies have found that cannabis users who drive while intoxicated double their risk of a car crash (Asbridge, Hayden & Cartwright, 2012). Evidence suggests that recent cannabis smoking is associated with substantial driving impairment, particularly in occasional smokers. The increased risk of motor vehicle accidents in these studies has persisted after statistical adjustment for confounding. For example, Mura et al. (2003) found an increased risk of accidents in a case-control study of 900 persons hospitalized in France with motor vehicle injuries and 900 age- and sex-matched controls admitted to the same hospitals for reasons other than trauma. Laumon and colleagues (2005) compared blood THC levels in 6766 culpable and 3006 non-culpable drivers in France between October 2001 and September 2003. Culpability was higher in drivers with THC levels greater than 1 ng/mL (OR = 2.87) and there was a dose–response relationship between blood THC and culpability that persisted after controlling for BAC, age and time of accident.

A meta-analysis of nine case-control and culpability studies (Asbridge, Hayden & Cartwright, 2012) found that recent cannabis use (indicated by either THC in blood or self-reported cannabis use) doubled the risk of a car crash (OR = 1.92, 95% CI: 1.35, 2.73). The risk was higher in better-designed studies (2.21 vs. 1.78), case-control rather than culpability studies (2.79 vs. 1.65) and studies of fatalities rather than injuries (2.10 vs. 1.74). Very similar results were reported in a meta-analysis by Li et al. (2012) (who reported a pooled risk estimate of 2.66) and in a systematic review of laboratory and epidemiological studies

(Hartman & Huestis, 2013). The risk of an accident increases substantially if cannabis users also have elevated blood alcohol levels, as many do (Hartman & Huestis, 2013).

Finally, a meta-analysis of 72 estimates of the risk of injury from cannabis was obtained from 46 studies, including some of the studies referred to above but also several others (Elvik, 2015). A random-effects model of analysis produced estimates of the risk of injury associated with the use of cannabis (95% confidence intervals in parentheses) and after adjustment for publication bias (Table 5.1).

Table 5.1. Estimates of the risk of injury associated with the use of cannabis

	Unadjusted	Adjusted for publication bias
Fatal injury	1.37 (1.24; 1.52)	1.37 (1.24, 1.51)
Serious injury	1.96 (1.27; 3.02)	1.84 (1.19, 2.85)
Other injury (severity not specified)	1.41 (0.97; 2.05)	1.12 (0.78, 1.62)
Property damage only	1.43 (1.26; 1.63)	1.11 (0.93, 1.32)

A test for publication bias suggested bias at all levels of injury severity, but not severe enough to influence the summary estimates of risk very much.

The analysis also found a relationship between the prevalence of cannabis use in drivers and the risk of injury associated with using cannabis. The fewer drivers that used cannabis, the higher the risk associated with its use. This pattern probably reflected selective recruitment of risky drivers to use cannabis.

The Driving Under the Influence of Drugs, Alcohol, and Medicines (DRUID) study was a population-based study of accident risks related to the use of cannabis and other drugs in nine EU countries (Hels et al., 2012). A pooled analysis found that drivers who tested positive for THC were 1–3 times more likely to be in an accident than sober drivers. This is comparable to a BAC level of 0.05 g/dl to <0.10 g/dl but the confidence intervals around these estimates were wide. A Department of Transportation case-control study in the USA found that drivers who tested positive for THC had 1.25 times higher risk of collision than a sober driver, but the association disappeared when age, gender, ethnicity and BAC levels were taken into account (Berning, Compton & Wochinger, 2015).

The existing evidence points to a small causal impact of cannabis on traffic injury. There are plausible biological pathways, and the pooling of studies found significant effects for cannabis. Overall, even though the effect is small compared to the effects of alcohol, traffic injury may be the most important adverse public health outcome for cannabis in terms of mortality in high-income countries (Fischer et al., 2015).

5.1.7 Other injury (not related to driving)

Some recent epidemiological studies of cannabis use and general injury risk have produced mixed findings. Gerberich and colleagues (2003) found that, among 64 657 patients in a health maintenance organization, cannabis users had higher rates of hospitalization for injury from all causes than former cannabis users or non-users. A meta-analysis of injury studies related to cocaine and cannabis users found that cannabis use was related to intentional injuries, as well as injuries in general, in cannabis-using clients of addiction treatment services (Macdonald et al., 2003). However, the authors argued that the evidence was not conclusive on the risk of injury among cannabis users. A Canadian survey study of 1999 adults who reported a history of traumatic brain injury had higher odds of reported past-year daily smoking (adjusted odds ratio [AOR] = 2.15), use of cannabis (AOR = 2.80) and use of nonmedical opioids (AOR = 2.90) (Ilie et al., 2015).

A case-crossover study among a sample of injured male and female patients in the emergency department in Lausanne, Switzerland, found that acute cannabis use (within a six-hour window) was associated with a reduced risk of injury (Gmel et al., 2009). The combined use of cannabis and alcohol was also not associated with an increased injury risk (Gmel et al., 2009). The authors suggested that the inconsistency between their findings and other studies could be explained by the fact that cannabis users in their study used cannabis at home whereas drinkers of alcohol usually consumed alcohol in bars where smoking cannabis did not frequently occur (Gmel et al., 2009). Another recent study among injured patients in the emergency department in Vancouver, Canada, also did not find an increased risk of injury associated with cannabis use. It did find, however, that the combined use of alcohol and drugs (with cannabis the most frequently reported drug) increased an individual's risk of being injured compared to non-drug-using controls (Cherpitel et al., 2012). Both studies used self-reported data on cannabis use prior to the injury and at the control time period.

5.1.8 Cannabis and the workplace

The effects of cannabis use on cognition in the context of work and everyday life, and whether off-site cannabis use endangers a worker or his colleagues while at work, are of concern (Phillips et al., 2015, Goldsmith et al., 2015). This topic has not been systematically investigated in recent years.

5.1.9 Areas that require more research

A. The epidemiological evidence on the effects of cannabis on driving is increasing but it is still small compared to evidence on the effects of alcohol.

- Larger and better-controlled studies are needed:
  - to clarify the magnitude of the risk of traffic injuries and to resolve inconsistent findings from recent studies (Berning, Compton & Wochinger, 2015);
  - on how tolerance may affect accident risk among regular cannabis users. Chronic heavy drinkers develop tolerance to alcohol and show fewer obvious signs of intoxication even at extremely high BAC levels. They can in many cases drive a

car with BAC levels at which others with a lower tolerance would not be able to drive (Chesher, Greeley, & Saunders, 1989).
- Differences in impairments for the same dose of THC also need to be investigated in naïve and experienced users (Berning, Compton & Wochinger, 2015).
- Studies are needed to investigate the effects of high THC levels on driving.
- Studies are required to compare the effects of smoking and of ingested cannabis on driving.

B. Some studies in the literature on driving use self-reported cannabis use as a marker.

- Future research should rely only on biological specimens which are more reliable markers of cannabis use. At least one report found inconsistencies between self-reported cannabis use and biological specimens collected from crash victims (Asbridge et al., 2014), though all measures showed elevated risk.

C. A number of developed countries have introduced roadside drug testing to deter drivers from driving while impaired by cannabis.

- Evaluations of the effectiveness of these countermeasures would provide some indication of the magnitude of the effect that cannabis use has on road crash risk (Hall, 2012).

D. Although a recent study found no increased risk of injury associated with cannabis use, which suggests that the setting in which cannabis is used may affect the risk (Gmel et al., 2009), other studies show the use of cannabis to be associated with increased injuries in adolescents and increased burns.

- Research is needed to understand the effect on injury risk of the social environment in which cannabis is typically consumed.

6. Mental health and psychosocial outcomes of long-term cannabis use

6.1 What do we know?

The adverse psychosocial and mental health outcomes that are correlated with long-term cannabis use are most often seen in daily or near-daily users. This section of the document summarizes evidence on the best researched of these health outcomes – namely dependence, educational outcomes, the use of other illicit drugs, cognitive impairment, mental disorders (psychoses, depression and other disorders) and suicidality (risk, ideation, attempts and mortality).

6.1.1 Long-term cannabis use and dependence

Cannabis dependence is a cluster of behavioural, cognitive and physiological phenomena that develop after repeated cannabis use. A diagnosis of dependence requires that three or more of the following criteria are met in the previous year:

(a) strong desire or sense of compulsion to take the substance;

(b) difficulties in controlling substance-taking behaviour in terms of its onset, termination, or levels of use;

(c) a physiological withdrawal state (see F1x.3 and F1x.4) when substance use has ceased or been reduced, as evidenced by: the characteristic withdrawal syndrome for the substance; or use of the same (or a closely related) substance with the intention of relieving or avoiding withdrawal symptoms;

(d) evidence of tolerance, such that increased doses of the psychoactive substances are required in order to achieve effects originally produced by lower doses (clear examples of this are found in alcohol- and opiate-dependent individuals who may take daily doses sufficient to incapacitate or kill nontolerant users);

(e) progressive neglect of alternative pleasures or interests because of psychoactive substance use, increased amount of time necessary to obtain or take the substance or to recover from its effects;

(f) persisting with substance use despite clear evidence of overtly harmful consequences, such as harm to the liver through excessive drinking, depressive mood states consequent to periods of heavy substance use, or drug-related impairment of cognitive functioning; efforts should be made to determine that the user was actually, or could be expected to be, aware of the nature and extent of the harm" (WHO, 1992).

Harmful use of cannabis and cannabis dependence are the most common forms of drug-use disorders in epidemiological surveys in Australia, Canada and the USA. These disorders affect 1–2% of adults in the past year, and 4–8% of adults during their lifetime (Hall & Pacula, 2010; Anthony, 2006). As noted, the risk of dependence has been estimated at 16% in those who initiated cannabis use in adolescence (Anthony, 2006) and 33–50% in daily cannabis users (van der Pol et al., 2013). We do not know how these risk estimates from the early 1990s may have been affected by changes in diagnostic criteria for dependence in DSM-5 or by changes in the potency of cannabis products. However, based on DSM-IV and the large representative USA NESARC study, higher proportions of lifetime users seem to have developed cannabis use disorders (Lev-Ran et al., 2013; Fischer et al., 2015), and nearly 3 of 10 cannabis users in the USA manifested a cannabis-use disorder in 2012–2013 (Hasin et al., 2015).

Humans develop tolerance to THC (Lichtman & Martin, 2005) and cannabis users who seek help for cannabis-use problems often report withdrawal symptoms such as anxiety, insomnia, appetite disturbance and depression (Budney & Hughes, 2006). These symptoms are of sufficient severity to impair everyday functioning (Allsop et al., 2012) and they are markedly attenuated by doses of an oral cannabis extract (Sativex) that contains THC (Allsop et al., 2014).

Cannabis dependence in and of itself is not the only problem for heavy users. By increasing the duration of regular use, dependence may also increase the risk of any long-term health risks of cannabis that may occur after decades of use, such as cardiovascular and respiratory diseases, and possibly cancers. These risks are discussed in chapter seven of the report.

The mortality of patients with cannabis dependence is also of concern. A study of 46 548 individuals hospitalized in California between 1990 and 2005 with ICD-9 diagnoses of cannabis dependence and cannabis abuse were followed for 16 years. Age-, sex- and race-adjusted standardized mortality rates (SMRs) were generated. Out of the total cohort of people with cannabis-use disorder diagnosis, 1809 deaths across all years were identified (Callaghan et al., 2012). This is an approximately four-fold higher risk of mortality when compared with that of the general population. The underlying reasons for the elevated standardized mortality rates in the cannabis cohort are unknown.

6.1.2 Long-term cannabis use and cognitive function

The 1990s case-control studies found that regular cannabis users had poorer cognitive performance than non-cannabis-using controls (Hall, Solowij & Lemon, 1994). The challenge was to decide whether cannabis use impaired cognitive performance, or if persons with poorer cognitive functioning were more likely to become regular cannabis users, or both (Hall, Solowij & Lemon, 1994). Better-controlled case-control studies since then (Crane et al., 2013; Solowij & Battisti, 2008; Grant et al., 2003; Schreiner & Dunne, 2012) have consistently found deficits in verbal learning, memory and attention in regular cannabis users (see section 5.1.2). These deficits have usually been correlated with the duration and frequency of cannabis use, the age of initiation and the estimated cumulative dose of THC (Solowij, 2002; Solowij & Pesa, 2012; Solowij et al., 2011). It remains unclear whether cognitive function fully recovers after cessation of cannabis use, with studies producing conflicting results (Solowij, 2002; Solowij & Pesa, 2012).

A longitudinal study from the Dunedin birth cohort suggested that sustained heavy cannabis use over several decades produced substantial declines in cognitive performance that may not be wholly reversible. This study assessed changes in IQ between age 13 (before cannabis was used) and at age 38 in 1037 New Zealanders born in 1972 or 1973 (Meier et al., 2012). Early and persistent cannabis users showed an average decline of eight IQ points compared with peers who had not used cannabis, and cannabis-using peers who had not used cannabis in this sustained way. Rogeberg (2013) argued that the apparent effect of sustained cannabis use on IQ could be due to failure to control for socioeconomic status. Further analysis of the Dunedin data did not support Rogeberg's hypothesis (Moffitt et al., 2013). A recent study in the USA has provided support for the study of Meier et al. in finding an association between poorer verbal memory and sustained daily use of cannabis throughout adult life (Auer et al., 2005).

As noted in section 4.1, studies of brain structure and function in cannabis users provide some support for these epidemiological findings. MRI studies have reported structural changes in the hippocampus, prefrontal cortex and cerebellum in chronic cannabis users

(Yücel et al., 2008) and these were largest in persons who had used cannabis the longest. A recent systematic review (Lorenzetti et al., 2013) found a consistent reduction in hippocampal volume in long-term daily users.

Excluding the possibility of reverse causation as an explanation for these findings has been difficult because younger persons with poorer cognitive performance are more likely to become regular cannabis users. There are also shared risk factors for regular cannabis use and poor cognitive performance. A causal role for regular cannabis use has biological plausibility in that cannabis acutely impairs cognitive performance, and neuroimaging studies have found relationships between the frequency and duration of cannabis use and structural and functional changes in brain regions implicated in memory and cognition.

6.1.3 Long-term psychosocial consequences of adolescent cannabis use

6.1.3.1 Social and educational outcomes

Longitudinal studies since the 1990s have found that cannabis use before the age of 15 years predicts early school-leaving and this persists after adjustment for confounders (e.g. (Ellickson et al., 1998)). A meta-analysis of three Australian and New Zealand longitudinal studies (Horwood et al., 2010) confirmed this finding. Longitudinal studies have also shown that early initiation of heavy cannabis use is associated with lower income, lower college degree completion, a greater need for economic assistance, unemployment, and use of other drugs (Fergusson et al., 2016; Fergusson & Boden, 2008; Brook et al., 2013).

It is plausible that educational outcomes in regular cannabis users are impaired for a combination of reasons: a higher pre-existing risk of educational problems in those who become regular cannabis users, the adverse effects of regular cannabis use on learning in school, increased affiliation of regular cannabis users with other cannabis-using peers who reject school, and the strong desire of younger cannabis users to make a premature transition to adulthood by leaving school (Lynskey & Hall, 2000).

A recent Australian twin study has raised doubts about a causal interpretation of the association between adolescent cannabis use and early school-leaving (Verweij et al., 2013). The study found that the association between early cannabis use and early school-leaving was explained by shared genetic and environmental risk factors. These findings have been supported by two twin studies in the USA (Grant et al., 2012; Bergen et al., 2008), which suggest that the association may be explained by higher levels of recruitment to cannabis use among adolescents who are at higher risk of leaving school earlier.

In an earlier Australian, study early-onset users had significantly higher rates of later substance use, juvenile offending, mental health problems, unemployment and school dropout. The links between early-onset cannabis use and later outcomes were largely explained by two routes that linked cannabis use to later adjustment. First, those electing to use cannabis were a high-risk population characterized by social disadvantage, childhood adversity, early-onset behavioural difficulties and adverse peer affiliations. Secondly, early-onset cannabis use was associated with subsequent affiliations with delinquent and substance-using peers, moving away from home and dropping out of education, with these factors in turn being associated with increased psychosocial risk (Fergusson et al., 1997). A substantial proportion of those who become cannabis users continued to smoke tobacco and use alcohol in a harmful or hazardous way and they were more likely to use a range of other illicit drugs (Hasin et al., 2015).

6.1.3.2 Other illicit drug use

Epidemiological studies in Australia, New Zealand and the USA in the 1970s and 1980s found that regular cannabis users were more likely to use heroin and cocaine, and that the younger they were when they first used cannabis the more likely they were to use the other drugs (Kandel, 2002). Three explanations were offered for these patterns: (a) that cannabis users had more opportunities to use other illicit drugs because these were supplied by the same black market as cannabis; (b) that early cannabis users were more likely to use other illicit drugs for reasons that were unrelated to their cannabis use (e.g. their propensity to take risks, behave impulsively, or engage in sensation-seeking); and (c) that the pharmacological effects of cannabis increased a young person's interest in using other illicit drugs (Hall & Pacula, 2010).

Patterns of drug involvement similar to those in the USA have been reported in a number of countries by epidemiological research (Swift et al., 2012), although the order in which drugs are used varies with the prevalence of different illicit drugs among adults (Degenhardt et al., 2010). Research has also supported the first two hypotheses in that young people in the USA who have used cannabis report more opportunities to use cocaine at an earlier age (Wagner & Anthony, 2002). Additionally, socially deviant young people (who are also more likely to use cocaine and heroin) start using cannabis at an earlier age than their peers (Fergusson, Boden & Horwood, 2008).

Simulations suggest that shared risk factors could explain these relationships between cannabis and other illicit drug use (Morral, McCaffrey & Paddock, 2002). The shared risk factor hypothesis has been tested in longitudinal studies by assessing whether cannabis users are more likely to report heroin and cocaine use after statistically controlling for confounding factors (Lessem et al., 2006; Fergusson, Boden & Horwood, 2006). Adjustment for confounders has reduced but not eliminated the relationship (Hall & Lynskey, 2005).

Studies of twins who are discordant for cannabis use (i.e. one used cannabis and the other did not) have been used to test whether shared genetic vulnerability explains the higher rates of illicit drug use among heavy cannabis users. Lynskey and colleagues (2003) found that the twin who had used cannabis prior to age 17 was more likely to have used other illicit drugs than the co-twin who had not. This relationship persisted after controlling for non-shared environmental factors. Similar results have been reported in discordant twin studies in the USA (Grant et al., 2010) and Netherlands (Lynskey, Vink & Boomsma, 2006).

Preclinical studies of early adolescent exposure to THC in rodents are supportive of these findings. Adult rats pre-treated with THC during adolescence and then allowed to mature to adults without THC are more likely to use heroin than rats not exposed to cannabis during adolescence. The endogenous opioid system was also disturbed in the brain of adults exposed to THC during adolescence (Ellgren, Spano & Hurd, 2007; Ellgren, 2008; Tomasiewicz et al., 2012).

6.1.3.3 Tobacco and alcohol use

In the early 1990s, cigarette smoking in many developed countries generally started before cannabis use, and regular tobacco smoking was a predictor of regular cannabis use and was regarded as a gateway to cannabis use. Over the past 20 years the relationship between cannabis and tobacco use has changed in some developed countries with a low prevalence of cigarette smoking and a high prevalence of cannabis use. In Australia and the USA, as a result of public health campaigns to prevent tobacco smoking among young people, young people increasingly start cannabis smoking before they smoke tobacco (Johnston et al., 2010). In these countries cannabis use increases the risk of becoming a tobacco smoker, a pattern described as a "reverse gateway" (Patton et al., 2005). Both gateway patterns probably reflect a shared route of administration (smoking) (Agrawal & Lynskey, 2009), the fact that cannabis smokers affiliate with tobacco smokers, and the effects of mixing tobacco and cannabis in joints.

In connection with the 2011 European School Survey Project on Alcohol and Other Drugs (ESPAD), a special study was undertaken on the prevalence of polydrug use among students from European countries that participated in the 2011 ESPAD survey (Hibell et al., 2012). Polydrug use was defined as the use of more than one of the following substances: tobacco (more than five cigarettes per day in the past 30 days), alcohol (consumption on 10 or more occasions in the past 30 days), cannabis (any use in the past 30 days), other illicit drugs (any lifetime use) and tranquillizers/sedatives without a prescription (any lifetime use). The overall prevalence of polydrug use (2-plus substances) in the total sample was very close to 9% in both survey years. The combination tobacco–cannabis was found in 9.7% of the polydrug group and the combination alcohol–cannabis was found in 5.7 %. The most common combination was tobacco–alcohol which was found in 12.4 % of the group (Hibell et al., 2012).

6.1.4 Psychosis and schizophrenia

In discussing relationships between cannabis use, psychosis and schizophrenia, it is necessary to define psychosis and schizophrenia clearly. Schizophrenia is a mental and behavioural disorder classified in the ICD-10. Schizophrenia is characterized by distortions in thinking, perception, emotions, language, sense of self and behaviour. Common experiences include hearing voices and delusions (WHO, 1992). Regular cannabis use has been reported to be more common among persons with schizophrenia (Myles, Myles & Large, 2015). The regular use of cannabis with a higher THC content and a lower CBD concentration may increase the risk for schizophrenia and lower the age of onset of the disease (Di Forti et al., 2014, 2015).

A 15-year follow-up study of schizophrenia among 50 465 Swedish male conscripts found that those conscripts who had tried cannabis by age the age of 18 years were 2.4 times more likely to be diagnosed with schizophrenia over the next 15 years than those who had not (Andréasson et al., 1987). After statistical adjustment for a personal history of psychiatric disorder by age 18 and a number of psychosocial confounders, those who had used cannabis 10 or more times by age 18 were 2.3 times more likely to be diagnosed with schizophrenia than those who had not used cannabis.

Zammit et al. (2002) reported a 27-year follow-up of the above-mentioned Swedish cohort. They also found a dose–response relationship between frequency of cannabis use at the age of 18 years and the risk of schizophrenia during the whole follow-up period (although the strength of the relationship declined with age). This effect persisted after statistically controlling for confounding factors. The researchers estimated that 13% of cases of schizophrenia would have been averted if no one in the cohort had used cannabis.

The Swedish cohort findings have been supported in smaller longitudinal studies in the Netherlands (van Os et al., 2002), Germany (Henquet et al., 2004) and New Zealand (Arseneault et al., 2002; Fergusson, Horwood & Swain-Campbell, 2003; Stefanis et al., 2014). All of these studies found a relationship between cannabis use and psychotic disorders or psychotic symptoms and these relationships persisted after adjustment for confounders. A meta-analysis of these longitudinal studies (Moore et al., 2007) reported that psychotic symptoms or psychotic disorders were higher in regular cannabis users than in non-users (OR 2.09 [95% CI: 1.54, 2.84]).

Reverse causation is a possible explanation of these findings if persons with schizophrenia use cannabis to relieve the symptoms of their illness. This possibility has been addressed to some extent in some of these longitudinal studies by excluding cases who reported psychotic symptoms at baseline, or by statistically adjusting for pre-existing psychotic symptoms. However, several large studies show that cannabis use preceded onset of psychosis (Andréasson et al., 1987; DiForti et al., 2009; Fergusson et al., 2003).

A second possibility is the common cause hypothesis – i.e. that the association is explained by other factors (e.g. genetic risk, childhood abuse) that increase the risk that young people will use cannabis and develop schizophrenia. This possibility has been addressed in some studies by comparing the rate of schizophrenia in persons who abuse different drugs. In a nationwide cohort of 30 547 patients receiving treatment for substance use disorders in Chile, there was an increased risk of a diagnosis of schizophrenia among cannabis users compared with patients who were users of other drugs (RR = 2.08, 1.6–2.7) and a dose–response association between cannabis use and risk of a schizophrenia diagnosis (Jorquera et al., 2015).

The common cause hypothesis has been harder to exclude because the association between cannabis use and psychosis is attenuated after statistical adjustment for potential confounders in many studies, and no study has been able to assess all plausible confounders. Genetic epidemiological studies have assessed the degree to which shared genetic risk factors may explain the association between cannabis use and psychoses. These have included studies of sib-pairs (McGrath et al., 2010), studies of the strength of the relationship between cannabis and psychosis in persons who differ in genetic relationship (Giordano et al., 2014), and correlations between polygenic risk scores for schizophrenia and cannabis use in large twin samples (Power et al., 2014). These studies suggest that shared genetic factors may explain some but not all of the association between cannabis and psychosis.

Researchers who favour a causal explanation point to its biological plausibility (e.g. (Di Forti et al., 2009)). This is indicated by double-blind studies which show that THC produces dose-related increases in positive and negative symptoms of psychosis in persons who do and do not have psychoses (D'Souza, 2004; Morrison, 2009; Murray et al., 2013). Psychotic syndromes have also been reported in patients who have been treated with the cannabinoid extract Sativex (Therapeutic Goods Administration, 2013). Compared with matched controls, those with psychotic disorders, and their siblings, are more sensitive to the psychotogenic effects of acute THC administration (D'Souza et al, 2005; Schizophrenia Working Group of the Psychiatric Genomics Consortium, 2014). A recent case-control study by Di Forti et al (2009) suggested that regular use of cannabis with high levels of THC and low levels of CBD increased the risk of developing schizophrenia by 3–5 times.

Researchers who remain sceptical about a causal role for cannabis (e.g. Gage, Zammit & Hickman, 2013) point to the absence of an increase in the incidence of schizophrenia as cannabis use increased among young adults. The evidence is mixed. An Australian modelling study did not find any marked increase in incidence after steep increases in cannabis use during the 1980s and 1990s (Degenhardt, Hall & Lynskey, 2003). However, a similar modelling study in the United Kingdom (Hickman et al., 2007) argued that it was too early to say. Two case register studies in Britain (Boydell et al., 2006) and Switzerland (Ajdacic-Gross et al., 2007) reported an increased incidence of psychoses in recent birth cohorts, but a United Kingdom study of general practice patients did not (Advisory Council on the Misuse of Drugs, 2008).

The available evidence points to a modest contributory causal role for cannabis in schizophrenia. There is a consistent dose–response relationship in a number of prospective studies between cannabis use in adolescence and the risk of developing psychotic symptoms or schizophrenia. Self-medication is implausible, and a causal relationship is biologically plausible (see Evins, in Haney & Evins, 2016). Researchers who are not convinced by the evidence argue that these studies have not excluded the possibility that the relationship is explained by residual confounding (see Haney, in Haney & Evins, 2016).

6.1.5 Other mental disorders

Depression is a common mental health problem and one of the most important contributors to the global burden of disease (Ustün et al., 2004; Moussavi et al., 2007). Findings of high prevalence of comorbid cannabis use and depression have been replicated in many large-scale cross-sectional studies and in mental health surveys. Persons with cannabis-use disorders have higher rates of depressive disorders (Swift, Hall & Teesson, 2001). In longitudinal studies, the relationship between regular cannabis use and depression has been much weaker than that for cannabis and psychosis (Degenhardt & Hall, 2012; Manrique-Garcia et al., 2012; Fergusson & Horwood, 1997). Meta-analyses of these studies (Moore et al., 2007) found modest associations between regular or heavy cannabis use and depressive disorders (Moore at al., 2007: OR = 1.49 [95% CI: 1.15, 1.94]; Lev-Ran et al., 2014: OR = 1.62 [95% CI 1.21-2.16]). Many of these studies did not adequately control for confounders, or excluded the possibility that depressed young people were more likely to use cannabis (Horwood et al., 2012) and in some studies associations disappear when better control is introduced (Feingold et al., 2015).

Much the same has been true of studies of cannabis-use disorders among persons diagnosed with bipolar disorders (e.g. (Lai & Sitharthan, 2012; Lev-Ran et al., 2013; Silberberg, Castle & Koethe, 2012; Agrawal, Nurnberger & Lynskey, 2011)). In one longitudinal study, cannabis use at baseline predicted an increased risk of manic symptoms in a three-year follow-up (Henquet et al., 2006). However, these studies have not adequately controlled for confounding variables or ruled out reverse causation with cannabis being used to lift depressed mood and reduce manic excitement (Silberberg, Castle & Koethe, 2012).

Persons with cannabis-use disorders also have higher rates of anxiety, conduct disorders, eating disorder and personality disorders (Goodman & George, 2015). The reasons for these common patterns of comorbidity have not been as well investigated in prospective studies as those between cannabis-use disorders and psychosis and depression. It remains to be discovered whether these disorders increase the risks of using cannabis (as is plausible for conduct and personality disorders), whether their outcomes are worsened by cannabis-use disorders, and to what degree these disorders share common risk factors with cannabis-use disorders (Hall, Degenhardt, & Teesson, 2009).

The high prevalence of comorbidity between drug-use disorders and other mental disorders does not mean that one causes the other, but comorbidity between mental and substance-use disorders is highly prevalent across countries. In general, people with a substance-use disorder had higher comorbid rates of mental disorders than vice versa, and people with drug-use disorders had the highest rates of comorbid mental disorders. In general, while there are associations between regular cannabis use or cannabis-use disorders and most mental disorders, causality has not been established. Reverse causation and shared risk factors cannot be ruled out as explanations of these relationships.

6.1.6 Suicide risk, ideation and attempts

Bagge and Borges (Bagge & Borges, 2015) conducted a case-crossover study of 363 persons who had recently attempted suicide and were treated in a trauma hospital for a suicide attempt within the previous 24 hours in the state of Mississippi, USA. The researchers compared rates of cannabis use in the 24 hours leading up to the suicide (case period) to that in the 24 hours of the day before the suicide (control period). They found that 10.2% of suicide attempters had used cannabis in the case period while 13.2% used cannabis in the control period.

The USA's Drug Abuse Warning Network (DAWN) estimated rates of cannabis use among drug-related visits to hospital emergency departments for suicide in 2011 (SAMHSA, 2013). Cannabis was coded as positive if hospital staff perceived it to be the cause or a contributor to the emergency visit. Cannabis was involved in an estimated 6.5% of drug-related suicide attempts, and in 46% of attempts the person also used alcohol. In the 23% of drug-related suicide attempts with toxicology reports, 16.8% tested positive for cannabis, although this cannabis use could have occurred days or even up to one week earlier. In general, 9.5% of all toxicology reports for deaths by suicide (Borges, Bagge & Orozco, 2016) show the presence of cannabis. There is preliminary evidence of higher detection of cannabis among suicide decedents that do not involve overdose (CDC, 2006) and higher detections among male suicide decedents using non-overdose methods than among females (Darke, Duflou & Torok, 2009; Shields et al., 2006). Homicide victims appear to have higher detection rates of cannabis at the time of death than suicide victims do (Darke, Duflou & Torok, 2009; Sheehan et al., 2013).

Overall, studies on cannabis use and suicide ideation and attempts have produce mixed results. A case-control study of 302 serious suicide attempts in New Zealand and general hospital community controls (Beautrais, Joyce & Mulder, 1999) found an association between harmful use of cannabis and suicide attempt. The association was substantially reduced after statistical adjustment for confounding. A small case-control study in the USA did not find an association (Petronis et al., 1990). Results from longitudinal studies are more numerous and have varied as to whether the associations persisted after adjustment for confounders, with newer and larger studies reporting positive associations. Fergusson and colleagues (Fergusson, Lynskey & Horwood, 1996; Fergusson & Horwood, 1997) found that regular cannabis use at the age of 15 years predicted ideation and attempts at 16–17 years in New Zealand, but these associations disappeared after controlling for confounders (Fergusson & Horwood, 1997). A 30-year follow-up of the cohort (van Ours et al., 2013) found a dose–response relation between cannabis use and suicidal ideation that persisted after controlling for confounding variables. The New Zealand Dunedin birth cohort (McGee, Williams & Nada-Raja, 2005) also reported an association between cannabis use at 15 years of age and suicidal ideation at 18–21 years of age, but this was no longer statistically significant after adjustment for confounders. A pooled analysis of Australian and New Zealand cohort studies found a dose–response relation between the frequency of cannabis use before the age of 17 years and suicide attempts at 17–25 years (Silins et al., 2014).

Longitudinal studies in the USA and other countries have found associations between cannabis use and suicidality over varying follow-up periods. In some studies the associations vary with age and the measure of cannabis use (e.g. Newcomb, Vargas-Carmona & Galaif, 1999; Newcomb, Scheier & Bentler, 1993). Others have found associations with suicidal ideation but not with suicide attempts (Juon & Ensminger, 1997). In some studies the association has persisted after controlling for confounding variables (e.g. Bovasso, 2001; Borowsky, Ireland & Resnick, 2001; Clarke et al, 2014; Pedersen, 2008), whereas in other studies it has not persisted, or has persisted only among subgroups (e.g. Wilcox & Anthony, 2004; Zhang & Wu, 2014; Wichstrom, 2000).

6.1.7 Suicide mortality

There have been very few studies of associations between regular cannabis use and death by suicide. A follow-up study of Swedish conscripts (Andréasson & Allebeck, 1990) reported that those who had used cannabis more than 50 times by the age of 18 years were at increased risk of dying by suicide. The same association was observed in a 33-year follow-up (Price, 2009) but it was no longer significant after adjusting for baseline alcohol, tobacco and other drug use, and psychiatric disorders.

A case-control study conducted among 108 individuals who committed suicide and 108 who died in accidents, matched for age and gender, in Cali, Colombia, found an increased odds ratio (OR=2.85(95% CI= 1.31–6.24) among those with cannabis-use disorders (Palacio et al., 2007). A large case-control study of 1463 suicides and 7392 natural deaths (Kung, 2003; Kung, 2005) found an association between any cannabis use and suicide risk after adjusting for depression, alcohol and mental health services. So did a four-year follow-up of a large group of patients with cannabis-use disorders in Denmark, which found an increased risk

(Males OR=2.28 (95% CI=1.54– 3.37); Females OR=4.82 (95% CI= 2.47–9.39))) of suicide among those with cannabis-use disorders (Arendt, 2013).

6.1.8 Areas that require more research

There have been recent reports that higher proportions of lifetime users seem to have developed cannabis-use disorders.

As a result, updated longitudinal research (including dose–response, potency, frequency of use, and age of onset and reason for use) is needed to identify if and why more users seem to develop cannabis-use disorders.

Better epidemiological and longitudinal studies are needed to determine the association between cannabis use and the risk of different types of mental disorders and suicidal ideation, attempts and death. These studies should include a wide age range, diverse social and geographical populations, and should better measure cannabis use in order to assess dose–response relations.

- Baseline measures should be chosen to rule out reverse causation and, if possible, third causes such as concurrent use of other substances, mental disorders and genetic vulnerability.
- Improved genetic studies are required to investigate the overlap between genotype and phenotype for schizophrenia and cannabis-use disorders.
- Persons with cannabis-use disorders have higher rates of depressive disorders. Many of these studies have not adequately controlled for confounders or excluded the possibility that depressed young people are more likely to use cannabis.
- Persons with cannabis-use disorders also have higher rates of anxiety, conduct disorders, eating disorder and personality disorders. The reasons for these common patterns of comorbidity have not been well investigated in prospective studies. Such investigation is needed.

While the evidence tends to suggest that cannabis use is associated with suicide ideation and suicidal behaviour, the lack of homogeneity in the measurement of cannabis exposure across studies and, in some instances, the lack of systematic control for known risk factors are clear limitations in current knowledge (Borges, Bagge & Orozco, 2016).

- Specifically for suicidal behaviour, efforts should be made to disentangle any effects of regular cannabis use from the short-term effects of use on suicidal ideation and behaviour.

7. Long-term cannabis use and noncommunicable diseases

7.1 What do we know?

7.1.1 Respiratory diseases

7.1.1.1 Chronic bronchitis

Considerable epidemiological and clinical research has assessed whether cannabis smoking is a risk factor for chronic obstructive pulmonary disease (COPD). The major symptoms of COPD are chronic bronchitis, chest tightness, increased cough and increased sputum most days of the year for two or more years. In most of these studies, cannabis-only smokers have been more likely to have reported cough, sputum and wheezing but no more likely to report shortness of breath than controls who do not smoke cannabis (Aldington et al., 2007; Bloom et al., 1987; Moore et al., 2005; Tan et al., 2009; Tashkin et al., 1987; Taylor et al., 2000).

In follow-up studies of habitual cannabis smokers, those who quit show reductions in cough, sputum and wheeze compared to those who continue to smoke cannabis. For example, a detailed analysis of a large, well-characterized cohort of nearly 1000 subjects followed from birth to age 38 years and assessed for respiratory symptoms at 18, 21, 26, 32 and 38 years, found strong associations between current cannabis use and morning cough, sputum production and wheeze over multiple assessments at different ages. Those who quit or very substantially reduced their cannabis smoking showed marked improvements in these symptoms (Hancox et al., 2015). Similar findings had been reported previously (Tashkin, Simmons & Tseng, 2012). Taken together, these and other findings suggest that the chronic bronchitis induced by cannabis smoke is reversible (Hancox et al., 2015; Tashkin, Simmons & Tseng, 2012).

A common finding in video bronchoscopy studies in cannabis-only smokers is swelling and oedema that blocks and partially occludes the bronchi (Roth, 1998). This is consistent with a modest increase in airway resistance that is of unclear clinical significance (Tashkin, 1987; Aldington, 2007; Hancox et al., 2010). Biopsies of bronchial mucosal tissue of cannabis-only smokers showed more replacement of the normal ciliated cells lining the airway with mucus-secreting and other cells than in nonsmokers (Roth et al., 1998; Fligiel et al., 1997). The reduction in ciliated cells, and subsequent increased mucus secretion from the larger number of mucus-secreting cells, probably explain the increased symptoms of chronic bronchitis in regular cannabis smokers (Tashkin, 2015).

7.1.1.2 Chronic obstructive pulmonary disease

COPD is a progressive disease that produces faster-than-normal annual age-related decreases in lung function in tobacco smokers. Studies have not found an increased risk of COPD in cannabis-only smokers. Chronic bronchitis occurs in the absence of COPD in most studies of cannabis smokers (e.g. Hancox et al., 2015; Kempker, Honig & Martin, 2015; Pletcher et al.,

2012; Sherrill et al., 1991; Tashkin et al., 1980; Taylor et al., 2000). No impairments in respiratory function were observed in three of the four longitudinal studies of lung function in regular cannabis smokers (Hancox et al., 2010; Pletcher et al., 2012; Tashkin et al., 1997). Although cannabis smokers do not appear to be at greater risk of COPD, they lose lung function more quickly than nonsmokers, even if the rate of decline is slower than that in tobacco smokers.

The only abnormality found in lung function tests was a modest increase in airway resistance (Tashkin et al., 1987; Aldington et al., 2007; Hancox et al., 2010), which is probably due to oedema in the airways of cannabis-only smokers. In some studies, cannabis smokers have had larger lung volumes than non-cannabis smokers, probably because the deep inhalations used in smoking cannabis stretch the lung (Tashkin, 2015).

Tobacco smoke activates alveolar macrophages, the major immune cell located in the lungs. These macrophages release cytokines and chemokines that stimulate the release of tissue-damaging products that can cause chronic bronchitis and emphysema. Cannabis smokers, in contrast to tobacco smokers, show reduced macrophage activity, presumably because of the immunosuppressive activity of THC (Tashkin, 2015).

7.1.1.3 Other respiratory diseases

There have been case reports of bullous lung disease (pathologically enlarged air spaces in the lung parenchyma measuring more than 1 cm) in cannabis smokers who use varying amounts of tobacco (Johnson, 2000; Phan, Lau & Li, 2005; Hii et al., 2008). This disease could compromise lung function and predispose to pneumothorax, but the causal relationship to cannabis is unclear (Tan, Hatam & Treasure, 2006).

Several cases of *Aspergillus* and other forms of pneumonia have also been reported in immunocompromised cannabis smokers (Tashkin, 2015). Cannabis smoking impairs the function of alveolar macrophages, key immune-effector cells in the lung's defence against infection (Baldwin et al., 1997). The loss of cilia and increased mucus-secreting cells in the airways of regular cannabis smokers (Fligiel et al., 1997) may impair mucociliary clearance, thereby increasing the risk of pneumonia. Cannabis use could predispose to pneumonia as a consequence of cannabis-related impairment in the lung's defences against infection. Since cannabis has also been shown to be frequently contaminated with *Aspergillus fumigatus* (Kagen, 1983) and potentially pathogenic gram-negative bacteria (Ungerleider, 1982), the introduction of these microorganisms into the lung by smoking provides an additional mechanism whereby cannabis could increase the risk of pneumonia. Well-designed epidemiological studies are needed to investigate this risk.

7.1.2 Cardiovascular diseases

One of the most reliable signs of cannabis intoxication is tachycardia or elevated heart rate (Chesher & Hall, 1999; Jones, 2002; Sidney, 2002). The CB_1 and CB_2 cannabinoid receptors are both found in the cardiovascular system (Montecucco & Di Marzo, 2012). Young daily cannabis users in laboratory studies develop tolerance to these effects within 2–4 weeks (Jones, 2002). Middle-aged men with a history of myocardial infarction who smoke cannabis can experience acute symptoms of angina; such cases were reported in the literature as early as in the 1970s (Gottschalk, Aronow & Prakash, 1977). Furthermore, cannabis has been shown to trigger, earlier than does tobacco, the occurrence of angina pectoris symptoms after physical effort among patients with a history of coronary disease or stable angina pectoris (Aronow & Cassidy, 1974).

There is a limited number of epidemiological studies of CVD in cannabis smokers (Sidney, 2002). Mittleman et al. (2001) found that the risk of myocardial infarction was four times higher in patients with a recent myocardial infarction in the hour after smoking cannabis, and then rapidly declined. The authors note that this risk was much less than that of cocaine (nearly 24 times in the first hour after use) (Mittleman et al., 1999).

A prospective study of 1913 adults found a dose–response relationship between cannabis use and cardiovascular mortality over 3.8 years (Mukamal et al., 2008). The risk was 2.5 times higher in those who used cannabis less than weekly and 4.2 times higher among those who used it weekly or more often. Cannabis use was not significantly associated with long-term mortality in patients from the same cohort after 18 years follow-up, although mortality rates were systematically higher in cannabis users than in non-users (Frost et al., 2013).

Recent case reports and case series suggest that cannabis smoking may increase the risk of CVD in younger cannabis smokers who are otherwise at relatively low risk (Arora et al., 2012; Bailly et al., 2010; Basnet, Mander & Nicolas 2009; Canga et al., 2011; Casier et al., 2014; Deharo, Massoure & Fourcade, 2013; Duchene et al., 2010; Hodcroft, Rossiter & Buch, 2014; Karabulut & Cakmak, 2010; Kocabay et al., 2009; Pratap & Korniyenko, 2012; Renard et al., 2012). Jouanjus et al (2014) reported that there were 35 cases of CVD in French cannabis users reported by health providers to the national Addictovigilance network between 2006 and 2010. These complications occurred in patients with a mean age of 34 years and, on the basis of their clinical history, could be attributed to cannabis use. The authors used capture-recapture measures to estimate the rate of reporting that resulted in 0.4% (Jouanjus et al., 2012). On the basis of this result, the 35 cases reported should be regarded as a considerable underestimate of the number of CVD that could have occurred among young cannabis users in France during the study period. During this study period, it is noteworthy that the portion of cannabis-related cardiovascular complications increased by a factor of three.

A third of cannabis-related hospitalizations in Toulouse, France, were attributed to CVD. These included seven myocardial infarctions, four cerebral strokes and three cases of juvenile thromboarteritis (Jouanjus et al., 2011). In another study of hospitalizations for CVD in young people (aged 15–30 years), cannabis was involved in 18 of 20 cases that involved a psychoactive drug. Many of these myocardial infarctions occurred in young cannabis users with few risk factors for CVD. Overall the data in the literature report that normal arteries were generally found in coronary angiographies, suggesting that vasospasm could be responsible for these events. Besides, cannabis smoking increases CVD risk by increasing carboxyhaemoglobin levels (Wu et al., 1988). As a result, the signal of an increasing risk of serious cannabis-related cardiovascular disorders was identified and confirmed in France. The cardiovascular complications observed in young cannabis users differed from those presented by non-using patients of the same age.

The impact of second-hand cannabis smoke on vascular endothelial function has recently begun to be discussed and examined. This research (Xiaoyin et al., 2014) concluded that cannabis and tobacco smoke impair endothelial function similarly under comparable exposure conditions. It also concluded, as have several other studies, that it is the smoke and not the THC that causes the impairment.

7.1.2.1 Stroke

In recent decades, the incidence of stroke in young adults has increased, as have case reports of stroke in cannabis smokers (Wolff et al., 2013). In 2013, Wolff found only 59 cases of cannabis-associated strokes in the literature. These were ischaemic strokes or transient ischaemic attacks that occurred in persons with a mean age of 33 years. By 2015, around 100 cases of cannabis-related ischaemic stroke had been reported (Wolff et al., 2013; Desbois & Cacoub, 2013; Hackam, 2015; Wolff et al., 2015). Some case-control studies also suggested that cannabis smoking was a risk factor for stroke in young adults (Barber et al., 2013), and at least five cases of ischaemic stroke have been reported in persons using synthetic cannabinoids (Benson-Leung, Leung & Kumar, 2013; Freeman et al., 2013; Takematsu et al., 2014).

Wolff (Wolff et al., 2011), for instance, described a 21-year-old male who had a cerebellar ischaemic stroke after smoking cannabis. Wolff argued that this stroke could be attributed to multifocal intracranial arterial stenosis because: (a) the patient had a normal cranial angiogram six months before he started smoking cannabis; (b) his cerebral arteries were stenosed at the time of the stroke; and (c) the stenoses were reversed after three months of abstinence from cannabis use. Cannabis-associated strokes usually occur in chronic or current cannabis users who smoke tobacco (Wolff et al., 2013). The stroke often occurs while the drug is being smoked, or minutes afterwards. There are several case reports of a recurrence of strokes in patients who did not stop using cannabis (Wolff et al., 2013). The cardiovascular effects of cannabis provide possible mechanisms for these strokes – namely, orthostatic hypotension, altered cerebral vasomotor function, supine hypertension and swings in blood pressure, cardio-embolism, vasculopathy, vasospasm and reversible vasoconstriction cerebral syndrome (Wolff et al., 2013). Furthermore, a French study of young adults (under the age of 45 years) who had an ischaemic stroke over a two-year period found that 13 of 48 were cannabis users. In 10 of the 13, the cause of stroke was multifocal intracranial arterial stenosis (Wolff et al., 2011). There was a reversal of cerebral vasoconstriction (documented by vascular imaging three months after diagnosis) in all patients who stopped using cannabis. This suggests that cannabis use can produce ischaemic stroke in young adults by inducing reversible cerebral vasoconstriction.

A five-year follow-up of cases of reversible cerebral vasoconstriction syndrome (RCVS) in 159 ischaemic strokes in young patients found RCVS to be the cause of 13% of these strokes, most often in men with a mean age of 32 years. In 67% of these cases the precipitant was smoking cannabis resin. The cerebral vasoconstriction resolved within 3–6 months if patients abstained from smoking cannabis (Wolff et al., 2015). The cerebral vasoconstriction induced by cannabis is a possible mechanism for these strokes (Wolff et al., 2015).

7.1.3 Cancer

THC and other cannabinoids are not carcinogens in microbial assays (MacPhee, 1999; Marselos & Karamanakos, 1999) or tests using rats and mice (Chan, 1996). However, cannabis smoke is carcinogenic in these assays (MacPhee, 1999; Marselos & Karamanakos, 1999; Leuchtenberger, 1983). This suggests that cannabis smoking could, like cigarette smoking, be a cause of cancers of the lung, the upper aerodigestive tract (mouth, tongue, oesophagus) and bladder (MacPhee, 1999). This could be true because there is a strong qualitative similarity between the carcinogens found in cannabis and tobacco smoke (Institute of Medicine, 1999; Van Hoozen & Cross, 1997). The existing case reports raise a suspicion, but provide limited support for the hypothesis, that cannabis use can cause upper respiratory tract cancers. The quality of the case reports is insufficient as they do not compare rates of cannabis use in cases and controls; rather, they assess cannabis exposure retrospectively, in the knowledge that the user has cancer, and they do not control for confounding factors such as alcohol and tobacco use (Hall et al., 2002).

7.1.3.1 Upper aerodigestive tract cancers

The evidence on the risks of upper area digestive tract cancers in cannabis smokers is not consistent. Two studies have shown an increased risk (Zhang et al., 1999; Feng et al., 2009), two have shown a decreased risk (Liang, 2009; Zhu et al., 2002), and five have found no association (Aldington et al., 2008a; Hashibe et al., 2006; Llewellyn, Johnson & Warnakulasuriya, 2004; Llewellyn et al., 2004; Rosenblatt et al., 2004). Pooled analyses have not found an overall association for head and neck cancer (Berthiller et al., 2008), but there is a possible increased risk of oropharyngeal cancer and a decreased risk of oral and tongue cancers (Marks et al., 2014). Three studies on the relationship between human papillomavirus (HPV) and cannabis and the risk of head and neck cancer suggest that HPV (which is a strong risk factor for oropharyngeal cancer) may be a modifying risk factor (Gillison et al., 2008; Liang et al., 2009; Marks et al., 2014). Future research on upper aerodigestive tract cancers needs to take into account the effects of concomitant alcohol and tobacco use as well as HPV infection.

7.1.3.2 Respiratory cancers

The Swedish conscript study (Callaghan, Allebeck & Sidorchuk, 2013) found a doubling of lung cancer rates among conscripts who had smoked cannabis 50 or more times by the age of 18 years. However, the study could control only for baseline tobacco use. Case-control studies of lung cancer in North Africa have found consistent associations but in all these studies cannabis smoking has been confounded by cigarette smoking (Mehra et al., 2006). A Tunisian case-control study of 110 cases of hospital-diagnosed lung cancer and 110 community controls found an association with cannabis use (OR = 8.2) that persisted after adjustment for cigarette smoking. A pooled analysis of three Moroccan case-control studies also found an elevated risk of lung cancer among cannabis smokers, but these cannabis users also smoked tobacco (Berthiller et al., 2008). A New Zealand case-control study of lung cancer in 79 adults under the age of 55 years and 324 community controls (Aldington et al., 2008b) found a dose–response relationship between frequency of cannabis use and lung cancer risk. Yet a collaborative pooled analysis of these epidemiological studies found no overall association between cannabis smoking and lung cancer and no evidence of a dose–response relationship (Zhang et al., 2015).

7.1.3.3 Testicular cancer

Three studies have found an association between cannabis smoking and testicular cancer. All are USA studies published since 2009. One of these, Daling et al. (2009), reported a case-control study of cannabis use among 369 men diagnosed with a testicular germ cell tumour and 979 age-matched controls. They found a higher rate of cannabis use among cases (OR = 1.7 [95% CI: 1.1, 2.5]). The risk was higher for a nonseminoma (OR = 2.3 [95% CI: 1.4, 4.0]) and was higher in those who used cannabis before the age of 18 years and used cannabis more often than weekly. These findings have since been replicated in two further case-control studies (Lacson et al., 2012; Trabert et al., 2011). Another case study published by of the University of Southern California in Los Angeles found that men with these tumours were about twice as likely to have a history of using cannabis.

A meta-analysis of these studies (Gurney et al., 2015) found an odds ratio of 1.5 for high frequency cannabis users and an odds ratio of 1.5 for those who had used cannabis for 10 or more years. This is a moderate and consistent relationship and, because tobacco smoking is not a cause of testicular cancer, there is no potential confounding by tobacco smoking. Cannabinoid receptors are found in the testes so a causal connection is not implausible.

7.1.3.4 Other cancers

With cannabis use, there is a trend towards increased prostate cancer (i.e. 3-fold risk), and cervical cancer (i.e. 1.4-fold risk). An elevated risk of prostate cancer was reported among cannabis smokers in an 8.6-year follow-up of 64 855 members of the Kaiser Permanente Medical Care Program (Sidney et al., 1997). Males who smoked cannabis had an increased risk of prostate cancer, as did males who were current cannabis smokers (Sidney et al., 1997). Confounding by other lifestyle factors was a possible explanation of the finding because AIDS-related deaths were higher among cannabis users in this study.

Smaller sized studies have implicated cannabis use in the development of bladder cancer and testicular germ cell tumours. The reasons for the great heterogeneity in epidemiological studies correlating cannabis use and cancer may be related to difficulties in quantifying cannabis use, unmeasured confounders in the cases or controls, and variable expression of cannabinoid receptors in target tissues.

Cannabis smoking during pregnancy has been associated with cancers among children. Three case-control studies for different cancers have found an association (Robinson et al., 1989; Grufferman, 1993; Kuijten, 1992). Each study examined cannabis use as one of many other risk factors for these cancers and there was no a priori reason to expect a relationship between cannabis use and the cancers. None of these results have been replicated. The incidence of these cancers did not increase over the period 1979–1995 in the USA when cannabis use was common (Reis et al., 2000; Smith et al., 2000; Gurney et al., 2000).

7.1.4 Areas that require more research

In view of the high prevalence of cannabis use worldwide, the French finding of an increasing risk of serious cannabis-related cardiovascular disorders should be explored in other countries.

Among the possible directions for future research are: a) to identify the mediators involved in the occurrence of the cardiovascular effects of cannabinoids; b) to assess the role of risk factors such as pre-existing CVD; and iii) to evaluate the potential therapeutic value of medical cannabinoids in preventing myocardial infarction.

- To collect more data on the increasing risk of CVD, health providers should be encouraged to investigate cannabis exposure systematically, including from second-hand smoke, in young patients presenting with cardiovascular disorders and patients receiving treatment with pharmaceutical preparations of cannabinoids.
- Better estimates of the rate of ischaemic stroke in young cannabis users are needed. Health providers should systematically asked about cannabis use, and especially the use of cannabis resin, when treating young patients with ischaemic stroke.
- More research is needed on the effects of cannabis on cerebral arteries in patients who develop a stroke. It is imperative that physicians ask young people with ischaemic strokes about their drug use, do arterial imaging to search for intracranial arterial stenosis, and evaluate the reversibility of the vascular abnormalities.
- Larger cohort and better designed case-control studies are needed to better control for the effects of cigarette smoking in order to clarify lung, head and neck, prostate and testicular cancer risks among long-term regular cannabis smokers (Hashibe et al., 2005).
- Future research on upper aerodigestive tract cancers needs to take into account the effects of concomitant alcohol and tobacco use as well as HPV infection.
- Studies are needed to compare the effects of smoking with vaporizing and ingestion of cannabis on the occurrence of cancer in various tissues, and to account for levels of THC and other cannabinoids.

Cannabis smoking impairs the function of alveolar macrophages, key immune-effector cells in the lung's defence against infection. The loss of cilia and increased mucus-secreting cells in the airways of regular cannabis smokers may impair mucociliary clearance and thereby increase the risk of pneumonia.

- Well-designed epidemiological studies are needed to investigate this risk and also the impact of cannabis smoking on persons other than the smoker (by environmental smoke).

8. Prevention and treatment

8.1 What do we know?

8.1.1 Prevention of cannabis use

There is emerging research on evidence-based prevention and increased knowledge on what is effective and what is necessary to implement and scale up preventive interventions. Most behavioural preventive interventions (environmental, universal, targeted and indicated approaches) have an impact on several problematic behaviours, including substance use (tobacco, alcohol, drugs and new psychoactive substances), and preventive interventions should cover the whole prevention chain from universal and selective to indicated prevention. This section of the document is limited to a short summary of those behavioural preventive interventions that are found to have a special beneficial or likely beneficial impact on cannabis use (in addition to other outcomes). Interventions aimed at reducing the harm associated with cannabis use by young people are included in section 8.1.2 on treatment. Widely adopted interventions without strong evidence of effectiveness, such as stand-alone media campaigns or information given alone to reduce drug use among young people (Ferri et al., 2013; Jepson et al, 2010), are not covered in this report.

8.1.1.1 Interventions targeting families

Family prevention strategies are thought to be "likely beneficial" (EMCDDA, 2013). A study of comprehensive family prevention that involved training for parents, children and the family collectively was found to be effective in reducing both lifetime cannabis use and past-year use in adolescents (Gates et al., 2006).

Furthermore, a Cochrane review of substance-use prevention found that family-based prevention programmes were more effective than youth-only programmes (Foxcroft & Tsertsvadze., 2011).There are additional encouraging results with regard to the long-term effects of family-based intervention on youth substance use (Foxcroft et al., 2014). Seven of eight family-based programmes examined in randomized controlled trials (six universal, two selective) showed positive effects during a period of at least two years (EMCDDA, 2015).

Some programmes provide adolescents or parents with services specific to their particular needs (Medina-Mora, 2005) and simultaneously address varying levels of risk (universal, selective and indicated) for both individual and family problems. A number of programmes of this kind have been tailored and tested, and those that have been evaluated have been found to have good results (Sanders, 1999). It may be less stigmatizing to reach these adolescents and families within universal-level prevention activities that target the whole population rather than in settings with more individually tailored intervention approaches (such as "programmes for families in need").

8.1.1.2 Interventions in school settings

Life skills programmes that combine both a social competence curriculum and social influence approaches have been shown to reduce cannabis use at 12-month follow-up and beyond, as compared to controls (Faggiano et al., 2005). This kind of school-based intervention includes social skills lessons and interpersonal rehearsals, activities to boost self-esteem, refusal skills, skills in recognizing high-risk situations, and normative educational methods. School-based social influence interventions alone have been found to be effective in reducing cannabis use in one randomized clinical trial (Faggiano et al., 2010).

Another review of school-based studies has found that interactive drug curricula are more effective than non-interactive, lecture-based drug curricula. Over 200 such studies found a delay in onset of substance use and a reduction in youth cannabis use (Tobler et al., 2000). Peer-led interventions using peer educators in school settings have also been shown to be effective in reducing all substance use in a systematic review (McGrath et al., 2006). However, this effect was reduced by the one- and two-year follow-up points.

A Cochrane review in 2014 concluded that programmes based on a combination of social competence and social influence approaches seemed to have better results than other types of approaches, with effective results in preventing cannabis use at longer follow-up, and in preventing any drug use. Knowledge-based interventions showed no differences in outcomes, apart from knowledge, which was improved among participants involved in the programmes (Fabbiano et al., 2014).

Effective classroom management is shown to create a positive school environment that can be a proactive way to prevent several problems – including early onset of cannabis use – while creating a positive learning environment.

8.1.1.3 Interventions targeting vulnerable youth

Interactive, social programmes targeting vulnerable young people have been found to be effective in reducing past-month cannabis use. Programmes that provide life skills development, team-building content, interpersonal communication skills, and introspective learning involving self-reflection were found to be effective in reducing cannabis use in high-risk youth (Springer et al., 2004).

Other comprehensive approaches that combine the involvement of community, school and family have been found to be effective in a systematic review (Jones et al., 2006). This combined effort reduced use, delayed use and prevented use among high-risk adolescents when compared to community-only or school-only programmes (Jones et al., 2006).

8.1.2 Treatment of disorders due to cannabis use

8.1.2.1 Natural history of cannabis-use disorders

For many young people cannabis use is time-limited; it is most common in persons in their early twenties and ceases in their late twenties (Hall & Degenhardt, 2015). The long-term frequent cannabis users who have tried and failed to stop are those most likely to have cannabis-use disorders and to seek help from treatment services. Many persons who meet the criteria for dependence cease their cannabis use without treatment and they no longer meet the criteria for dependence when followed up a few years later. In Australia, the Victorian Adolescent Cohort Study, which tracked individuals dependent on cannabis for four years, found that more than half of those that initially met dependence criteria no longer did so after four years (Coffey et al., 2003). In a German study, over 80% of individuals who met criteria for dependence at an initial assessment were "in remission" at 10 years follow-up (Perkonigg et al., 2008).

8.1.2.2 Therapies for cannabis-use disorders

Brief psychological interventions based on motivational interviewing techniques have been shown to increase rates of cannabis cessation at 3 months (RR 3.33 [95% CI 1.99 to 5.56]) and at 8–12 months (RR 2.41 [95% CI 1.01 to 5.73]) (NCCMH, 2008). While this evidence has been used to promote very brief (as short as 5 minutes) opportunistic interventions in primary care settings, the trials identified in this review used trained psychologists to deliver interventions lasting 30–60 minutes.

While effective for harmful cannabis use, single-session interventions are of limited value in the treatment of cannabis dependence. A recent review by WHO found evidence from clinical trials to support the use of several approaches for the treatment of cannabis dependence, including combinations of measures to increase motivation (with motivational enhanced therapy [MET], cognitive-behavioural therapy [CBT] and contingency management [CM] providing specific rewards), together with family therapy interventions in adolescents (WHO, 2015).

CBT, MET and a combination of CBT, MET and psychosocial problem-solving therapy (PPS) were more effective than a waiting list control. CBT and MET produced a 50% reduction in continuous measures of cannabis use and were equally efficacious in head-to-head trials. For adolescents with cannabis dependence, family interventions were more effective than individual counselling in producing abstinence, and family and social interventions were more effective than psychoeducation alone.

An EMCDDA systematic review found similar results (EMCDDA, 2015). CBT and multidimensional family therapy, a type of family therapy, were found to reduce cannabis use moderately in adolescent users. MET/CBT combined with CM has also been shown to improve abstinence rates in this group. In contrast to the WHO review, MET alone produced results similar in effect to psychoeducation. Similarly, in the EMCDDA review of treatments for adult users, CBT and motivational interviewing (MI) in combination were found to be helpful, with MI alone producing a small effect (EMCDDA, 2015). In a review of trials which included patients with different substance-use disorders, keeping in mind that cannabis is the most commonly cited drug for treatment entry, family-based interventions – specifically BSFT, MI and CBT – were found to induce small but significant reductions in use (EMCDDA, 2015).

No medications have been found to be effective for treating cannabis dependence. A Cochrane review published in 2014 (Marshall et al., 2014) found that antidepressants, bupropion, buspirone and atomoxetine were ineffective, and that evidence was lacking for other potential therapeutic medications such as THC, gabapentin and N-acetylcysteine.

8.1.2.3 Management of acute cannabis intoxication and cannabis withdrawal

Various medications have been used to manage the acute effects of cannabis, such as anxiety, tachycardia, arrhythmias and psychotic symptoms. These medications include beta-blockers, antiarrhythmic agents, antagonists of CB-1 receptors and GABA-benzodiazepine receptors, antipsychotics and cannabidiol. Propranol, rimonabant, flecainidine, propafenone, flumazenil, olanzapine and haloperidol have all been used in the management of cannabis intoxication. There is a lack of data on the comparative effectiveness of different compounds in management of many of the acute presentations of cannabis intoxication; however, beta-blockers do reduce the tachycardia and hypertension associated with cannabis intoxication. It is likely that benzodiazepines will reduce anxiety in cannabis-induced panic disorders, although this has not been specifically tested (Crippa et al., 2012).

Arrhythmias from cannabis intoxication can be normalized by using antiarrythmic agents such as flecainide, propafenone and digoxin (Rubio et al., 1993; Kosior et al., 2001; Fisher et al., 2005). Flumazenil, an antagonist of the GABA-benzodiazepine receptor complex, has been effective in treating cannabis-induced comatose states that are fortunately very rare and typically occur when children accidentally ingest cannabis products (Crippa et al., 2012). Haloperidol and olanzapine have been found to be effective in reducing psychotic symptoms (Berk et al., 1999). Cannabidiol, a component of cannabis that does not produce psychoactive effects, has been shown to reduce anxious and psychotic symptoms induced by THC (Zuardi et al., 1982).

Different medications were evaluated in the management of cannabis withdrawal, including lithium (Winstock et al., 2009), lofexidine (Haney et al., 2008), nefazodone and bupropion (Carpenter et al., 2009) and, more recently, agonists of cannabinoid receptors such as dronabinol and nabiximols with encouraging results (Allsop et al., 2014; Allsop et al., 2015). However, the effectiveness of these medications in the management of cannabis withdrawal is not yet well established.

8.1.2.4 Relapse prevention

As with other substance-use disorders, relapse after cessation of cannabis use is common. To reduce the chances of relapsing to cannabis use and dependence, attention to the risk and protective factors associated with drug use may be useful. Risk factors for adolescents include conflict in the family and friends who use cannabis. Protective factors in adolescence include a positive relationship with parents, which provides structure and boundaries, a positive school environment, and engagement in activities that provide meaning (WHO, 2001). Protective factors in adulthood include employment, housing and social support. Risk factors include untreated mental health conditions.

8.1.3 Areas that require more research

- The adverse health and social consequences of cannabis use reported by cannabis users who seek treatment for dependence are less severe than those reported by alcohol- and opioid-dependent persons (Hall & Pacula, 2010; Degenhardt, 2012). However, rates of recovery from cannabis dependence among those seeking treatment are similar to those for alcohol dependence (Florez-Salamanca et al., 2013). Clinical trials of cognitive behaviour therapy for cannabis dependence show that only a minority remain abstinent 6–12 months after treatment. Nonetheless, treatment substantially reduces the severity of cannabis-related problems and the frequency of cannabis use (Roffman, 2006; Danovitch, 2012).

- Evidence on the effectiveness of telephone and Internet interventions is limited, although some reviews have reported reductions in cannabis use. This is an area for future research. These interventions may be of particular value in individuals who recognize that they have a problem with cannabis use but are not ready to enter an addiction treatment programme. This approach is also a cheaper option for countries with limited resources.
- Few studies analyse the fidelity of the implementation of different psychological interventions so it is difficult to know with certainty that the interventions are the same across various countries or even various treatment centres within the same country.

9. Conclusions

9.1 What do we know?

In summary there is less knowledge about the health and social effects of nonmedical cannabis use than about the use of alcohol and tobacco. On the basis of the current review by experts, the following conclusions of the known and unknown effects can be made.

9.1.1 What do we know about the neurobiology of cannabis use?

We know the following:

- CB1 receptors (which respond to THC) are widely distributed in the brain, including areas that control attention, decision-making, motivation and memory.
- These receptors modulate the effects of a variety of other neurotransmitter systems.
- Short-term and long-term cannabis use down-regulates these receptors in ways that may explain the short-term and long-term effects of cannabis on working memory, planning and decision-making, response speed, accuracy and latency motivation, motor coordination, mood and cognition.

9.1.2 What do we know about the epidemiology of cannabis use and cannabis dependence?

We know the following:

- Cannabis is the most widely used illicit drug globally. In 2013, an estimated 181.8 million people aged 15–64 years used cannabis for nonmedical purposes globally (uncertainty estimates 128.5–232.1 million).
- Cannabis use appears to be more common in developed countries than in developing countries, although we lack good data on prevalence of use in the latter.
- Young people often use cannabis, with the mid-teens being the age of first use in many developed countries.
- There has been an upward trend in the mean THC content of all confiscated cannabis preparations in the USA and some European countries.
- Cannabis dependence exists and is a cluster of behavioural, cognitive and physiological phenomena that develop after repeated cannabis use. There are some indications that the prevalence of cannabis dependence increased worldwide between 2001 and 2010.
- There is a major demand for addiction treatment systems for cannabis-use disorders in many high-income countries and in some low- and middle-income ones.

9.1.3 What do we know about the short-term effects of cannabis use?

We know the following:

The most obvious short-term health effect of cannabis is intoxication marked by disturbances in the level of consciousness, cognition, perception, affect or behaviour, and other psychophysiological functions and responses.

- A minority of first-time cannabis users become very anxious, have panic attacks, experience hallucinations and vomit. These symptoms may be sufficiently distressing to prompt affected users to seek medical care.
- Acute use impairs driving and contributes to an increased risk of traffic injuries.
- There is some evidence that cannabis use can trigger coronary events. Recent case reports and case series suggest that cannabis smoking may increase CVD risk in younger cannabis smokers who are otherwise at relatively low risk.

9.1.4 What do we know about the long-term effects of regular cannabis use?

We know the following:

- Regular cannabis users can develop dependence on the drug. The risk may be around 1 in 10 among those who ever use cannabis, 1 in 6 among adolescent users, and 1 in 3 among daily users.
- Withdrawal syndrome is well documented in cannabis dependence.
- Growing evidence reveals that regular, heavy cannabis use during adolescence is associated with more severe and persistent negative outcomes than use during adulthood.
- In a number of prospective studies there is a consistent dose–response relationship between cannabis use in adolescence and the risk of developing psychotic symptoms or schizophrenia.
- The association between cannabis use and psychosis or schizophrenia has been recognized for over two decades in at least four ways:
    1. Cannabis produces a full range of transient schizophrenia-like positive, negative and cognitive symptoms in some healthy individuals.
    2. In those harbouring a psychotic disorder, cannabis may exacerbate symptoms, trigger relapse and have negative consequences on the course of the illness.
    3. With heavy cannabis use, susceptible individuals in the general population develop a psychotic illness which is associated with age of onset of use, strength of THC in the cannabis, frequency of use and duration of use.
    4. Cannabis use is associated with lowering the age of onset of schizophrenia It is likely that cannabis exposure is a "component cause" that interacts with other factors to precipitate schizophrenia or a psychotic disorder, but is neither necessary nor sufficient to do so alone. Symptoms of schizophrenia increase with cannabis use and strength. The magnitude of the symptoms is associated with the amount used and the frequency of use. Daily use in adolescence and young adulthood is associated with a variety of negative health and psychological outcomes. These include:

- early school-leaving
- cognitive impairment
- increased risk of using other illicit drugs
- increased risk of depressive symptoms
- increased rates of suicidal ideation and behaviour.

It remains to be determined which of these associations are causal.
- Long-term cannabis smoking produces symptoms of chronic and acute bronchitis, as well as microscopic injury to bronchial lining cells, but it does not appear to produce COPD.
- Long-term heavy cannabis smoking can potentially trigger myocardial infarctions and strokes in young cannabis users.
- Smoking a mix of cannabis and tobacco may increase the risk of cancer and other respiratory diseases but it has been difficult to decide whether cannabis smokers have a higher risk, over and above that of tobacco smokers.
- There is suggestive evidence that testicular cancer is linked to cannabis smoking and this potential link should be investigated further.

9.1.5 What do we know about prevention and treatment?

We know the following:

- Evidence-based preventive interventions should cover the whole prevention chain from universal and selective to indicated prevention.
- Comprehensive family prevention that involves training for parents, children and the family collectively is found to be effective in reducing both lifetime cannabis use and past-year use in adolescents.
- Life skills programmes that combine both a social competence curriculum and social influence approaches are shown to reduce cannabis use at 12-month follow-up and beyond.
- Interactive social programmes targeting vulnerable young people is found to be effective in reducing past-month cannabis use.
- A single-session brief psychological intervention of 30–45 minutes increases the chances of cannabis cessation if people are not dependent on cannabis.
- Many people with cannabis-use disorders cease cannabis use without treatment.
- For people who are dependent on cannabis, family interventions are effective for adolescents, and CBT, MET and PPS are effective in adults.

9.2 Priority areas for future research

One of the objectives of the expert meeting held in 2015 was to identify areas for future research to enable us to learn more about both the association with and causality of cannabis use and health and social consequences. The areas identified by the experts were as follows 9.2.1–9.2.6).

9.2.1 Substance content and prevalence

We need to know more about:

- the THC content of cannabis products used by most cannabis users in different countries;
- the typical dose of THC received by regular cannabis users, and whether users titrate their dose of THC when using more potent cannabis products;
- whether increased rates of treatment-seeking are influenced by higher THC content in cannabis, whether cannabis products with higher THC content affect the adverse health effects of cannabis use, and whether increased THC content has been accompanied by a reduction in the CBD content of cannabis products;
- the prevalence of use in many low- and middle-income countries;
- the extent to which household and school surveys reach all cannabis users;
- global data on the prevalence of harmful patterns of cannabis use;
- the prevalence of changing routes of cannabis administration (e.g. use of vaporisers and edible cannabis products);
- the global prevalence of heavy cannabis use and cannabis-use disorders.

9.2.2 Neurobiology of cannabis use

We need to know more about:

- the extent to which neurobiological changes and especially cognitive impairments are reversible in heavy cannabis users;
- the duration of acute impairments produced by cannabis (the length of time after using cannabis that psychomotor and cognitive performance are impaired);
- the possible results of longitudinal studies combining epidemiological and neuroimaging methods to study the effects of cannabis use on brain functioning;
- the possible replicability of neuroimaging studies of cannabis users by using standardized imaging methods, better statistical analyses and larger samples;
- whether genetics explain the observation that persons who score higher on sensation-seeking, aggression and antisocial behaviour have increased risks of cannabis-use disorder?

9.2.3 Health consequences

We need to know more about:

- case-control studies on the effects of cannabis use on motor vehicle accidents, and the relationship between cannabis use and other types of injury;
- how tolerance to cannabis in regular users affects the ability to drive;
- the triggering effects of cannabis on coronary heart events, especially myocardial infarction;
- the effects of cannabis use during pregnancy or conception through investigations using better methods of assessing cannabis use;
- the effects of regular long-term cannabis use on various cancer risks, specifically

- – upper aerodigestive tract cancers, while taking into account the effects of concomitant alcohol and tobacco use,
  - – respiratory cancers that better control for the effects of tobacco smoking,
  - – head and neck cancers that stratify for HPV status;
- in countries with a high prevalence of cannabis use, the link between cannabis smoking and CVD in young adults, specifically
  - – cardiac syndromes and infarctions,
  - – strokes and cerebral ischaemic events;
- the potentially causal effects of long-term cannabis use on the risks of mental disorders, specifically
  - – psychoses and particularly schizophrenia,
  - – major depression and bipolar disorders,
  - – anxiety disorders;
- the effects of acute and regular cannabis use on suicide ideation, suicide attempts and death by suicide, while examining dose–response relations and controlling for other drug use.

9.2.4 Social costs

We need to know more about:

- epidemiological estimates of the social and economic costs of cannabis use.

9.2.5 Prevention

We need to know more about:

- the effect of preventive programmes for children of cannabis-affected families (as a result of more longitudinal research);
- how best to scale up prevention, targeting persons of different age groups and in different settings;
- what works in indicated prevention.

9.2.6 Treatment

We need to know more about:

- the effectiveness and cost-effectiveness of screening and brief interventions for hazardous and harmful cannabis use, including in educational settings;
- the effectiveness and cost-effectiveness of mobile telephone and Internet-based interventions for cannabis-use disorders;
- the effectiveness and cost-effectiveness of family interventions for cannabis-use disorders;
- potential effective pharmacotherapy for cannabis-use disorders.

References

Chapter 1

Global Burden of Disease Study 2013 Collaborators (2015). Global Burden of Diseases, Injuries, and Risk Factors Study 2013. Lancet. 386;9995:743–800.

Madras BK (2015). Update of cannabis and its medical use. Report to the WHO Expert Committee on Drug Dependence (http://www.who.int/medicines/access/controlled-substances/6_2_cannabis_update.pdf?ua=1, accessed 16 February 2016).

UNODC (2015). World drug report 2015. Vienna: United Nations Office on Drugs and Crime.

WHO (1997). Cannabis: a health perspective and research agenda. Geneva: World Health Organization:46.

WHO (2015). WHO Expert Committee on Drug Dependence: thirty-seventh report. Geneva: World Health Organization (in press).

Chapter 2

Ahmed SA, Ross SA, Slade D, Radwan MM, Zulfiqar F, Matsumoto RR, et al. (2008). Cannabinoid ester constituents from high-potency Cannabis sativa. J Nat Prod. 71(4):536–42.

APA (2013). Diagnostic and statistical manual of mental Disorders, fifth edition. Arlington (VA): American Psychiatric Association.

Azorlosa JL, Greenwald MK, Stitzer ML (1995). Marijuana smoking: effects of varying puff volume and breathhold duration. J Pharmacol Exp Ther. 272(2):560–9.

Azorlosa JL, Heishman SJ, Stitzer ML, Mahaffey JM (1992). Marijuana smoking: Effect of varying delta-9-tetrahydrocannabinol content and number of puffs. J Pharmacol Exp Ther. 261(1):114–22.

Bloor RN, Wang TS, Spanel P, Smith D (2008). Ammonia release from heated 'street' cannabis leaf and its potential toxic effects on cannabis users. Addiction. 103(10):1671–7.

Brands B, Sproule B, Marshman J, editors (1998). Drugs & drug abuse, third edition. Toronto: Addiction Research Foundation.

Bruci Z, Papoutsis I, Athanaselis S, Nikolaou P, Pazari E, Spiliopoulou C, et al. (2012). First systematic evaluation of the potency of Cannabis sativa plants grown in Albania. Forensic Sci Int. 222(1–3):40–6.

Cannon DS, Clark LA, Leeka JK, Keefe CK (1993). A reanalysis of the Tridimensional Personality Questionnaire (TPQ) and its relation to Cloninger's Type 2 Alcoholism. Psychol Assessment. 5:62–6.

Coffey C, Carlin JB, Lynskey M, Li N, Patton GC (2003). Adolescent precursors of cannabis dependence: Findings from the Victorian Adolescent Health Cohort Study. Brit J Psychiat. 182:330–6.

Collins D, Abadi MH, Johnson K, Shamblen S, Thompson K (2011). Non-medical use of prescription drugs among youth in an Appalachian population: prevalence, predictors, and implications for prevention. J Drug Educ. 41(3):309–26.

Costello EJ, Angold A (2011). Causal thinking in developmental disorders. In: Shrout PE, Keyes KM, Ornstein K, editors. Causality and Psychopathology: finding the determinants of disorders and their cures. Oxford: University Press:279–96.

Daniel JZ, Hickman M, Macleod J, Wiles N, Lingford-Hughes A, Farrell M, et al. (2009). Is socioeconomic status in early life associated with drug use? A systematic review of the evidence. Drug Alcohol Rev. 28(2):142–53.

Davy Smith G (2011). Obtaining robust causal evidence from observational studies: Can genetic epidemiology help? In: Shrout PE, Keyes KM, Ornstein K, editors. Causality and psychopathology: finding the determinants of disorders and their cures. Oxford: University Press:206–51.

Degenhardt L, Dierker L, Chiu WT, Medina-Mora, ME, Neumark Y, Sampson N, et al. (2010). Evaluating the drug use "gateway" theory using cross-national data: consistency and associations of the order of initiation of drug use among participants in the WHO World Mental Health Surveys. Drug and Alcohol Depen. 108(1–2):84–97.

Eisenberg E, Ogintz M, Almog S (2014). The pharmacokinetics, efficacy, safety, and ease of use of a novel portable metered-dose cannabis inhaler in patients with chronic neuropathic pain: a phase 1a study. J Pain Palliat Care Pharmacother. 28(3): 216–25.

ElSohly MA, Ross SA, Mehmedic Z, Arafat R, Yi B, Banahan BF (2000). Potency trends of delta(9)-THC and other cannabinoids in confiscated marijuana from 1980–1997. J Forensic Sci. 45(1):24–30.

Elsohly MA, Slade D (2005). Chemical constituents of marijuana: the complex mixture of natural cannabinoids. Life Sci. 78(5):539–48.

EMCDDA (2004). EMCDDA insights: an overview of cannabis potency in Europe. Luxembourg: Office for Official Publications of the European Communities.

EMCDDA (2015a). European drug report 2015: trends and developments. Lisbon: European Monitoring Centre for Drugs and Drug Addiction (http://www.emcdda.europa.eu/edr2015, accessed 8 August 2015).

EMCDDA (2015b). EMCDDA perspectives on drugs, new developments in Europe's cannabis market. Lisbon: European Monitoring Centre for Drugs and Drug Addiction.

Fehr K, Kalant H, editors (1983). Cannabis and health hazards: proceedings of an ARF/WHO scientific meeting on adverse health and behavioral consequences of cannabis use. Toronto: Addiction Research Foundation.Fergusson DM, Horwood LJ, Lynskey MT (1994). Parental separation, adolescent psychopathology, and problem behaviors. J Am Acad Child Psy. 33(8):1122–31.

Fergusson DM, Horwood LJ, Beautrais AL (2003). Cannabis and educational achievement. Addiction. 98(12):1681–92.

Fergusson D, Horwood L, Swain-Campbell N (2003). Cannabis dependence and psychotic symptoms in young people. Psychol Med. 33:15–21.

Fergusson D, Boden J, Horwood L (2008). The developmental antecedents of illicit drug use: evidence from a 25-year longitudinal study. Drug Alcohol Depend. 96(1-2):165–77.

Fergusson DM, Boden J, Horwood L (2015). Psychosocial sequelae of cannabis use and implications for policy: findings from the Christchurch Health and Development Study. Soc Psychiatry Psychiatr Epidemiol. 50:1317–26.

Gaoni Y, Mechoulam R (1964). Isolation, structure and partial synthesis of an active constituent of hashish. J Am Chem Soc. 86:1646–7.

Gerra G, Angioni L, Zaimovic A, Moi G, Bussandri M, Bertacca S, et al. (2004). Substance use among high school students: relationships with temperament, personality traits, and parental care perceptions. Subst Use Misuse. 39(2):345–67.

Gloss D (2015). An overview of products and bias in research. Neurotherapeutics. 12(4):731-4.

Hall WD, Degenhardt L (2007). Prevalence and correlates of cannabis use in developed and developing countries. Curr Opin Psychiatry. 20(4):393–7.

Hall W, Degenhardt L, Teesson M (2009). Understanding comorbidity between substance use, anxiety and affective disorders: broadening the research base. Addict Behav. 34:526–30.

Hall WD, Pacula RL (2010). Cannabis use and dependence: public health and public policy (reissue of first edition 2003). Cambridge: Cambridge University Press.

Hall WD (2015). What has epidemiological research revealed about the adverse health effects of cannabis in the past 20 years? Addiction. 110:19–35.

Hawkins J, Catalano R, Miller J (1992). Risk and protective factors for alcohol and other drug problems in adolescence and early adulthood: implications for substance abuse prevention. Psychol Bull. 112:64–105.

Hoch E, Bonnet U, Thomasius R, Ganszer F, Havemann-Reinecke U, Preuus UW (2015). Risks associated with non-medical use of cannabis. Dtsch Arztebl Int [German Medical Journal International]. 112:271–8.

Hill A (1965). The Environment and Disease: Association or Causation? Proc R Soc Med. May; 58(5): 295–300.PMCID: PMC1898525.

Iversen L (2007). The science of marijuana, second edition. Oxford: Oxford University Press.

Izzo AA, Borrelli F, Capasso R, Di Marzo V, Mechoulam R (2009). Non-psychotropic plant cannabinoids: new therapeutic opportunities from an ancient herb. Trends Pharmacol Sci. 30(10):515–27.

Kandel DB, Andrews K (1987). Processes of adolescent socialisation by parents and peers. Int J Addict. 22:319–42.

Kandel D (1993). Social demography of drug use. In: Bayer R, Oppenheimer GM, editors. Drug policy, illicit drugs in a free society. Cambridge: Cambridge University Press:24–77.

Kendler K, Chen X, Dick D, Maes H, Gillespie N, Neale MC, et al. (2012). Recent advances in the genetic epidemiology and molecular genetics of substance use disorders. Nat Neurosci. 15:181–9.

King KM, Chassin L (2004). Mediating and moderated effects of adolescent behavioral under control and parenting in the prediction of drug use disorders in emerging adulthood. Psychol Addict Behav. 18:239–49.

Korhonen T, Huizink AC, Dick DM, Pulkkinen L, Rose RJ, Kapiro J (2008). Role of individual, peer and family factors in the use of cannabis and other illicit drugs: a longitudinal analysis among Finnish adolescent twins. Drug Alcohol Depend. 97(1–2):33–43.

Lascala E, Friesthler B, Gruenwald PJ (2005). Population ecologies of drug use, drinking and related problems. In: Stockwell T, Gruenwald PJ, Toumbourou JW, et al., editors. Preventing harmful substance use: the evidence base for policy and practice. Chichester: John Wiley & Sons.

Lipkus IM, Barefoot JC, Williams RB, Siegler IC (1994). Personality measures as predictors of smoking initiation and cessation in the UNC Alumni Heart Study. Health Psychol. 13(2):149–55.

Lopez-Quintero C, Pérez de los Cobos J, Hasin DS, Okuda M, Wang S, Grant BF, et al. (2011). Probability and predictors of transition from first use to dependence on nicotine, alcohol, cannabis, and cocaine: results of the National Epidemiologic Survey on Alcohol and Related Conditions (NESARC). Drug Alcohol Depend. 115(1–2):120–30.

Lynskey M, Hall W (2000). The effects of adolescent cannabis use on educational attainment: a review. Addiction. 95(11):1621–30.

Lynskey MT, Fergusson DM, Horwood LJ (1994). The effect of parental alcohol problems on rates of adolescent psychiatric disorders. Addiction. 89(10):1277–86.

Lynskey MT, Fergusson DM (1995). Childhood conduct problems and attention deficit behaviors and adolescent alcohol, tobacco and illicit drug use. J Abnorm Child Psych. 23:281–302.Martin B, Cone E (1999). Chemistry and pharmacology of cannabis. In: Kalant H, Corrigal W, Hall W, et al., editors. The health effects of cannabis. Toronto: Centre for Addiction and Mental Health:19–68.

Mechoulam R, Hanus L (2012). Other cannabinoids. In: Castle D, Murray RM, D'Souza DC, editors. Marijuana and madness, second edition. Cambridge: Cambridge University Press:17-22.

Mednick SC, Christakis NA, Fowler JH (2010). The spread of sleep loss influences drug use in adolescent social networks. PLoS One. 5(3):e9775.

Mehmedic Z, Chandra S, Slade D, Denham H, Foster S, Patel AS, et al. (2010). Potency trends of Delta9-THC and other cannabinoids in confiscated cannabis preparations from 1993 to 2008. J Forensic Sci. 55(5):1209–17.

Moffat AC, Osselton MD, Widdop B, editors (2004). Clarke's analysis of drugs and poisons, third edition. Volume 2:743.London: Pharmaceutical Press.

Niesink RJ, Rigter S, Koeter MW, Brunt TM (2015). Potency trends of Δ(9)-tetrahydrocannabinol, cannabidiol and cannabinol in cannabis in the Netherlands: 2005–15. Addiction. 110(12):1941–50.

ONDCP (2007). Study finds highest levels of THC in U.S. marijuana to date. News release. Washington (DC): Office of National Drug Control Policy.

Pinchevsky GM, Arria AM, Caldeira KM, Garnier-Dykstra LM, Vincent KB, O'Grady KE (2012). Marijuana exposure opportunity and initiation during college: parent and peer influences. Prev Sci. 13:43–54.

Radwan MM, Elsohly MA, Slade D, Ahmed SA, Wilson L, El-Alfy AT, et al. (2008). Non-cannabinoid constituents from a high potency Cannabis sativa variety. Phytochemistry. 69(14): 2627–33.

Radwan MM, ElSohly MA, El-Alfy AT, Ahmed SA, Slade D, Husni AS, et al. (2015). Isolation and pharmacological evaluation of minor cannabinoids from high-potency Cannabis sativa. J Nat Prod. 78(6):1271–6.

Richmond RC, Al-Amin A, Smith GD, Relton CL (2014). Approaches for drawing causal inferences from epidemiological birth cohorts: a review. Early Hum Dev. 90(11):769–80.

Schulenberg JE, Merline AC, Johnston LD, O'Malley PM, Bachman JG, Laetz VB (2005). Trajectories of marijuana use during the transition to adulthood: the big picture based on national panel data. J of Drug Issues. 35:255–80.

Stone AL, Becker LG, Huber AM, Catalano RF (2012). Review of risk and protective factors of substance use and problem use in emerging adulthood. Addict Behav. 37:747–75.

Swift W, Wong A, Li KM, Arnold JC, McGregor IS (2013). Analysis of cannabis seizures in NSW, Australia: cannabis potency and cannabinoid profile. PLoS One. 8(7):e70052.

Townsend L, Flisher AJ, King G (2007). A systematic review of the relationship between high school dropout and substance use. Clin Child Fam Psychol Rev. 10(4):295–317.

Tu AW, Ratner PA, Johnson JL (2008). Gender differences in the correlates of adolescents' cannabis use. Subst Use Misuse. 43(10):1438–63.

UNODC (2015). World drug report 2015. Vienna: United Nations Office on Drugs and Crime.

von Sydow K, Lieb R, Pfister H, Höfler M, Wittchen HU (2002). What predicts incident use of cannabis and progression to abuse and dependence? A 4-year prospective examination of risk factors in a community sample of adolescents and young adults. Drug Alcohol Depend. 68(1):49–64.

Wilsey B, Marcotte T, Deutsch R, Gouaux B, Sakai S, Donaghe H (2013). Low-dose vaporized cannabis significantly improves neuropathic pain. J Pain. 14(2):136–48.

WHO (1992). The ICD-10 classification of mental and behavioural disorders. Clinical descriptions and diagnostic guidelines. Geneva: World Health Organization.

WHO (1993). The ICD-10 classification of mental and behavioural disorders. Diagnostic criteria for research. Geneva: World Health Organization.

Wymbs BT, McCarty CA, King KM, McCauley E, Vander Stoep A, Baer JS, et al. (2012). Callous-unemotional traits as unique prospective risk factors for substance use in early adolescent boys and girls. J Abnorm Child Psych. 40(7):1099–110.

Zamengo L, Frison G, Bettin C, Sciarrone R (2014). Variability of cannabis potency in the Venice area (Italy): a survey over the period 2010-2012. Drug Test Anal. 6(1–2):46–51.

Chapter 3

Anthony J, Warner L, Kessler R (1994). Comparative epidemiology of dependence on tobacco, alcohol, controlled substances and inhalants: basic findings from the National Comorbidity Survey. Exp and Clin Psychopharm. 2(3):244–68.

Anthony JC (2006). The epidemiology of cannabis dependence. In: Roffman RA, Stephens RS, editors. Cannabis dependence: its nature, consequences and treatment. Cambridge: Cambridge University Press:58–105.

Bhana A (2015). Adolescent cannabis use in Africa [background paper submitted to the WHO Scientific Meeting on Harms to Health Due to Cannabis, Stockholm, 21-23 April 2015].

Calabria B, Degenhardt L, Briegleb C, Vos T, Hall W, Lysneky M, et al. (2010). Systematic reviews of prospective studies investigating "remission" from amphetamine, cannabis, cocaine and opioid dependence. Addict Behav. 35:741–9.

Castillo Carniglia A (2015). Large increase in adolescent marijuana use in Chile. Addiction. 110(1):185–6.

Chopra RN, Chopra GS, Chopra IC (1942). Cannabis sativa in relation to mental diseases and crime in India. Indian J Med Res. 30:155–71.

Comisión Interamericanana para el Control del Abuso de Drogas (CICAD) (Inter-American Drug Abuse Control Commission) (2015). Informe sobre uso de drogas en las Américas 2015. Washington (DC): CICAD (www.cicad.oas.org/apps/Document.aspx?Id=3209, accessed 05 September 2015).

Compton WM, Grant BF, Colliver JD, Glantz MD, Stinson FS (2004). Prevalence of marijuana use disorders in the United States: 1991–1992 and 2001–2002. JAMA. 291(17):2114–21.

Cooper ZD, Haney M (2014). Investigation of sex-dependent effects of cannabis in daily cannabis smokers. Drug Alcohol Depend. 136:85–91.

Davis JM, Mendelson B, Berkes JJ, Suleta K, Corsi KF, Booth RE (2015). Public health effects of medical marijuana legalization in Colorado. Am J Prev Med. doi:10.1016/j.amepre.2015.06.034 (Epub ahead of print).

Degenhardt L, Hall WD (2012). Extent of illicit drug use and dependence, and their contribution to the global burden of disease. Lancet. 379(9810):55–70.

Degenhardt L, Ferrari AJ, Calabria B, Hall WD, Norman R, McGrath J, et al. (2013). The global epidemiology and contribution of cannabis use and dependence to the global burden of disease: results from the GBD 2010 Study. PLoS One. 8(10):e76635.

Dines AM, Wood DM, Galicia M, Yates CM, Heyerdahl F, Hovda KE, et al. (2015a). Presentations to the emergency department following cannabis use – a multi-centre case series from ten European countries. J Med Toxicol. 11(4):415–21.

Dines AM, Wood DM, Yates C, Heyerdahl F, Hovda KE, Giraudon I, et al. (2015b). Acute recreational drug and new psychoactive substance toxicity in Europe: 12 months data collection from the European Drug Emergencies Network (Euro-DEN). Clin Toxicol. 53(9):893–900.

El Omari F, Toufiq J (2015). The Mediterranean School Survey Project on Alcohol and Other Drugs in Morocco. Addicta. 2:30–9.

EMCDDA (2014). European Drug Report 2014: trends and developments [online publication]. Luxembourg: Publications Office of the European Union (www.emcdda.europa.eu/attachements.cfm/att_228272_EN_TDAT14001ENN.pdf, accessed 05 September 2015).

EMCDDA (2015a). European Drug Report 2015: trends and developments [online publication]. Luxembourg: Publications Office of the European Union (http://www.emcdda.europa.eu/edr2015, accessed 05 September 2015).

EMCDDA (2015b). EMCDDA Perspectives on Drugs: new developments in Europe's cannabis market. Lisbon, European Monitoring Centre for Drugs and Drug Addiction.

EMCDDA (2015c). Statistical bulletin [online publication]. Lisbon: European Monitoring Centre for Drugs and Drug Addiction (http://www.emcdda.europa.eu/data/stats2015, accessed 05 September 2015).

Hall WD, Pacula RL (2010). Cannabis use and dependence: public health and public policy, (reissue of first edition 2003). Cambridge: Cambridge University Press.

Hall WD (2015). What has epidemiological research revealed about the adverse health effects of cannabis in the past 20 years? Addiction. 110:19–35.

Hasin DS, Saha TD, Kerridge BT, Goldstein RB, Chou SP, Zhang H, et al. (2015). Prevalence of marijuana use disorders in the United States between 2001–2002 and 2012–2013. JAMA Psychiatry. 72(12):1235–42.

Horta RL, Horta BL, da Costa AW, do Prado RR, Oliveira-Campos M, Malta DC (2014). Lifetime use of illicit drugs and associated factors among Brazilian schoolchildren, National Adolescent School-based Health Survey (PeNSE 2012). Rev Bras Epidemiol [Brazilian Journal of Epidemiology]. 17:31–45.

Jungerman FS, Menezes PR, Pinsky I, Zaleski M, Caetano R, Laranjeira R (2009). Prevalence of cannabis use in Brazil: data from the I Brazilian National Alcohol Survey (BNAS). Addict Behav. 35(3):190–3. doi:10.1016/j.addbeh.2009.09.022.

Kaar SJ, Gao CX, Lloyd B, Smith K, Lubman DI (2015). Trends in cannabis-related ambulance presentations from 2000 to 2013 in Melbourne, Australia. Drug Alcohol Depend. 155:24–30.

Kadri N, Agoub M, Assouab F, Tazi MA, Didouh A, Stewart R, et al. (2010). Moroccan national study on prevalence of mental disorders: a community-based epidemiological study. Acta Psychiatrica Scandinavica. 122:340.

Liakoni E, Dolder PC, Rentsch K, Liechti ME (2015). Acute health problems due to recreational drug use in patients presenting to an urban emergency department in Switzerland. Swiss Med Wkly. 145:w14166.

NACADA (2007). Rapid assessment of drug and substance abuse in Kenya. Nairobi: National Authority for the Campaign Against Drug Abuse (http://www.nacada.go.ke/wp-content/uploads/2010/06/rapidassessment-web.pdf, accessed 6 September 2015).

NACADA (2012). Rapid assessment of drug and substance abuse in Kenya. Nairobi: National Authority for the Campaign Against Drug Abuse.

NIH (2012). National Epidemiologic Survey on Alcohol and Related Conditions-III (NESARC-III). Bethesda: National Institutes of Health.

SAMHSA (2012). Drug Abuse Warning Network (DAWN) 2010: national estimates of drug related emergency department visits. HHS publication no. (SMA)12-4733, DAWN series D-38. Rockville (MD): Substance Abuse and Mental Health Services Administration.

SAMHSA (2013). Drug Abuse Warning Network (DAWN) 2011: national estimates of drug related emergency department visits. HHS publication no. (SMA)13-4760, DAWN Series D-39. Rockville (MD): Substance Abuse and Mental Health Services Administration.

SENDA (2013). Décimo estudio nacional de drogas en población general de Chile 2012 [tenth national study of drugs in the general population of Chile]. Santiago: Servicio Nacional para la Prevención y Rehabilitación del Consumo de Droga y Alcohol; Observatorio Chileno de Drogas. (http://www.senda.gob.cl/wpcontent/uploads/2011/04/2012_Decimo_EstudioNacional.pdf, accessed 18 August 2015).

SENDA (2014). Décimo estudio nacional de drogas en población escolar de Chile 2013 [tenth national study of drugs in the school population of Chile]. Santiago: Servicio Nacional para la Prevención y Rehabilitación del Consumo de Droga y Alcohol ; Observatorio Chileno de Drogas.

SENDA (2015). Décimo primer estudio nacional de drogas en población general de Chile [eleventh national study of drugs in the general population of Chile]. Santiago: : Servicio Nacional para la Prevención y Rehabilitación del Consumo de Droga y Alcohol; Observatorio Chileno de Drogas (http://www.senda.gob.cl/media/2015/08/Informe-Ejecutivo-ENPG-2014.pdf, accessed 18 August 2015).

Roxburgh A, Hall WD, Degenhardt L, Mclaren J, Black E, Copeland J, et al. (2010). The epidemiology of cannabis use and cannabis-related harm in Australia 1993–2007. Addiction. 105(6):1071–9.

Smith DE (1968). Acute and chronic toxicity of marijuana. J Psychedelic Drugs. 2:37–47.

Thomas H (1993). Psychiatric symptoms in cannabis users. Brit J Psychiat. 163:141–9.

UNIAD/INPAD (2012). Unidade de pesquisas em álcool e drogas/Instituto nacional de ciència e tecnologia para políticas públicas do álcool e outras drogas. LENAD II (Levantamento Nacional de Álcool e Drogas II [Second national survey of alcohol and drugs]). São Paulo: Universidade federal de São Paulo (http://inpad.org.br/wp-content/uploads/2014/03/Lenad-II-Relat%C3%B3rio.pdf, accessed 05 September 2015).

UNODC (2015). World drug report 2015. Vienna: United Nations Office on Drugs and Crime.

Weil A (1970). Adverse reactions to marijuana, classification, and suggested treatment. NEJM. 282:997–1000.

WHO (2010). ATLAS on substance use (2010): resources for the preventions and treatment of substance use disorders. Geneva: World Health Organization.

Chapter 4

Anthony JC (2006). The epidemiology of cannabis dependence. In: Roffman RA, Stephens RS, editors. Cannabis dependence: its nature, consequences and treatment. Cambridge: Cambridge University Press:58–105.

Ashtari M, Avants B, Cyckowski L, Cervellione KL, Roofeh D, Cook P, et al. (2011). Medial temporal structures and memory functions in adolescents with heavy cannabis use. J Psychiat Res. 45(8):1055–66.

Batalla A, Bhattacharyya S, Yücel M, Fusar-Poli P, Crippa JA, Nogué S, et al. (2013). Structural and functional imaging studies in chronic cannabis users: a systematic review of adolescent and adult findings. PLoS One. 8(2):e55821. doi:10.1371/journal.pone.0055821.

Bidwell LC, Metrik J, McGeary J, Palmer RH, Francazio S, Knopik VS (2013). Impulsivity, variation in the cannabinoid receptor (CNR1) and fatty acid amide hydrolase (FAAH) genes, and marijuana-related problems. J Stud Alcohol Drugs. 74(6):867–78.

Bloomfield MA, Morgan CJ, Egerton A, Kapur S, Curran HV, Howes OD (2014). Dopaminergic function in cannabis users and its relationship to cannabis-induced psychotic symptoms. Biol Psychiatry. 75(6):470–8.

Bossong MG, Jager G, Bhattacharyya S, Allen P (2014). Acute and non-acute effects of cannabis on human memory function: a critical review of neuroimaging studies. Curr Pharm Des. 20(13):2114–25.

Cascio MG, Pertwee RG (2012). The function of the endocannabinoid system. In: Castle D, Murray R, D'Souza DC, editors. Marijuana and madness. Cambridge: Cambridge University Press:23–34.

Cheetham A, Allen NB, Whittle S, Simmons JG, Yücel M, Lubman DI (2012). Orbitofrontal volumes in early adolescence predict initiation of cannabis use: a 4-year longitudinal and prospective study. Biol Psychiatry. 71(8):684–92.

Churchwell JC, Lopez-Larson M, Yurgelun-Todd DA (2010). Altered frontal cortical volume and decision making in adolescent cannabis users. Front Psychol. 14(1):225.

Cousijn J, Wiers RW, Ridderinkhof KR, van den Brink W, Veltman DJ, Goudriaan AE (2012). Grey matter alterations associated with cannabis use: results of a VBM study in heavy cannabis users and healthy controls. Neuroimage. 59(4):3845–51.

Crean RD, Crane NA, Mason BJ (2011). An evidence based review of acute and long-term effects of cannabis use on executive cognitive functions. J Addict Med. 5(1):1–8.

Creemers HE, Buil JM, van Lier PA, Keijsers L, Meeus W, Koot HM, et al. (2015). Early onset of cannabis use: does personality modify the relation with changes in perceived parental involvement? Drug Alcohol Depend. 146:61–7. doi: 10.1016/j.drugalcdep.2014.11.004.

Danielsson AK, Falkstedt D, Hemmingsson T, Allebeck P, Agardh E (2015). Cannabis use among Swedish men in adolescence and the risk of adverse life course outcomes: results from a 20 year-follow-up study. Addiction. 10(11):1794–802. doi:10.1111/add.13042.

Day NL, Leech SL, Goldschmidt L (2011). The effects of prenatal marijuana exposure on delinquent behaviors are mediated by measures of neurocognitive functioning. Neurotoxicol Teratol. 33(1):129–36.

Di Forti M, Sallis H, Allegri F, Trotta A, Ferraro L, Stilo SA, et al. (2014). Daily use, especially of high-potency cannabis, drives the earlier onset of psychosis in cannabis users. Schizophr Bull. 40(6):1509–17.

DiNieri JA, Hurd YL (2012). Rat models of prenatal and adolescent cannabis exposure. Methods Mol Biol. 829:231–42.

DiNieri JA, Wang X, Szutorisz H, Spano SM, Kaur J, Casaccia P, et al. (2011). Maternal cannabis use alters ventral striatal dopamine D2 gene regulation in the offspring. Biol Psychiatry. 70(8):763–9.

EMCDDA (2015a). European Drug Report 2015: trends and developments. Lisbon: European Monitoring Centre for Drugs and Drug Addiction (http://www.emcdda.europa.eu/edr2015, accessed 05 September 2015).

EMCDDA (2015b). EMCDDA perspectives on drugs, new developments in Europe's cannabis market. Lisbon: European Monitoring Centre for Drugs and Drug Addiction.

Fried P, Watkinson B, Gray R (2005). Neurocognitive consequences of marijuana – a comparison with pre-drug performance. Neurotoxicol Teratol. 27(2):231–9.

Gerra G, Zaimovic A, Castaldini L, Garofano L, Manfredini M, Somaini L, et al. (2010). Relevance of perceived childhood neglect, 5-HTT gene variants and hypothalamus-pituitary-adrenal axis dysregulation to substance abuse susceptibility. Am J Med Genet B Neuropsychiatr Genet. 153B(3):715–22.

Goldschmidt L, Day NL, Richardson GA (2000). Effects of prenatal marijuana exposure on child behavior problems at age 10. Neurotoxicol Teratol. 22(3):325–36.

Goldschmidt L, Richardson GA, Cornelius MD, Day NL (2004). Prenatal marijuana and alcohol exposure and academic achievement at age 10. Neurotoxicol Teratol. 26(4):521–32.

Goldschmidt L, Richardson GA, Willford J, Day NL (2008). Prenatal marijuana exposure and intelligence test performance at age 6. J Am Acad Child Psy. 47(3):254–63.

Gruber SA, Sagar KA, Dahlgren MK, Racine M, Lukas SE (2012). Age of onset of marijuana use and executive function. Psychol Addict Behav. 26(3):496.

Hall WD (2015). What has epidemiological research revealed about the adverse health effects of cannabis in the past 20 years? Addiction. 110:19–35.

Hartman RL, Huestis MA (2013). Cannabis effects on driving skills. Clin Chem. 59(3):478-92. doi:10.1373/clinchem.2012.194381.

Hayatbakhsh MR, Najman JM, Bor W, O'Callaghan MJ, Williams GM (2009). Multiple risk factor model predicting cannabis use and use disorders: a longitudinal study. Am J Drug Alcohol Abuse. 35(6):399–407.

Hu SS, Mackie K (2015). Distribution of the endocannabinoid system in the central nervous system. In: Pertwee RG, editor. Handbook of Experimental Pharmacology. New York (NY): Springer:231:59–93.

Huestis MA, Gorelick DA, Heishman SJ, Preston KL, Nelson RA, Moolchan ET, et al. (2001). Blockade of effects of smoked marijuana by the CB1-selective cannabinoid receptor antagonist SR141716. Arch Gen Psychiatry. 58(4):322–8.

Iversen L (2012). How cannabis works in the human brain. In: Castle D, Murray R, D'Souza DC, editors. Marijuana and madness. Cambridge, Cambridge University Press:1–11.

Jacobus J, Tapert SF (2014). Effects of cannabis on the adolescent brain. Curr Pharm Des. 20(13):2186–93.

Konijnenberg C (2015). Methodological Issues in Assessing the Impact of Prenatal Drug Exposure. Substance;9(Suppl 2):39-44. PMID: 26604776.

Lopez-Larson MP, Bogorodzki P, Rogowska J, McGlade E, King JB, Terry J, et al. (2011). Altered prefrontal and insular cortical thickness in adolescent marijuana users. Behav Brain Res. 220(1):164–172.

Lopez-Larson MP, Rogowska J, Yurgelun-Todd D (2015). Aberrant orbitofrontal connectivity in marijuana smoking adolescents. Dev Cogn Neurosci. 16:54–62.

Lorenzetti V, Solowij N, Whittle S, Fornito A, Lubman DI, Pantelis C et al. (2015). Gross morphological brain changes with chronic, heavy cannabis use. Br J Psychiatry. 206(1):77–8.

Lorenzetti V, Solowij N, Fornito A, Lubman DI, Yücel M (2014). The association between regular cannabis exposure and alterations of human brain morphology: an updated review of the literature. Curr Pharm Des. 20(13):2138–67.

Lorenzetti V, Lubman DI, Fornito A, Whittle S, Takagi MJ, Solowij N, et al. (2013). The impact of regular cannabis use on the human brain: a review of structural neuroimaging studies. In: Miller PM, editor. Biological research on addiction. San Diego (CA): Academic Press: 711–28.

Mackie K (2005). Distribution of cannabinoid receptors in the central and peripheral nervous system. Handb Exp Pharmacol. (168):299–325.

Madras BK (2015). Update of cannabis and its medical use. Report to the WHO Expert Committee on Drug Dependence (http://www.who.int/medicines/access/controlled-substances/6_2_cannabis_update.pdf?ua=1 , accessed 16 February 2016).

Matochik JA, Eldreth DA, Cadet JL, Bolla KI (2005). Altered brain tissue composition in heavy marijuana users. Drug Alcohol Depend. 77(1):23–30.

Meier MH, Caspi A, Ambler A, Harrington H, Houts R, Keefe RS, et al. (2012). Persistent cannabis users show neuropsychological decline from childhood to midlife. Proc Natl Acad Sci U S A, 109(40):E2657–64.

Mena I, Dörr A, Viani S, Neubauer S, Gorostegui ME, Dörr MP (2013). Efectos del consumo de marihuana en escolares sobre funciones cerebrales demostrados mediante pruebas neuropsicológicas e imágenes de neuro-SPECT [Effects of consuming marijuana on school students' brain functions demonstrated through neuropsychological testing and neuro-SPECT imaging]. Salud mental. 36:367–74.

Moffitt TE, Meier MH, Caspi A, Poulton R (2013). Reply to Rogeberg and Daly: no evidence that socioeconomic status or personality differences confound the association between cannabis use and IQ decline. Proc Natl Acad Sci U S A. 110(11):E980–2.

Muro I, Rodríguez A (2015). Age, sex and personality in early cannabis use. Eur Psychiatry. 30(4):469–73.

Noland JS, Singer LT, Short EJ, Minnes S, Arendt RE, Kirchner HL, et al. (2005). Prenatal drug exposure and selective attention in preschoolers. Neurotoxicol Teratol. 27(3):429–38.

Pistis M, Perra S, Pillolla G, Melis M, Muntoni AL, Gessa GL (2004). Adolescent exposure to cannabinoids induces long-lasting changes in the response to drugs of abuse of rat midbrain dopamine neurons. Biol Psychiatry. 56(2):86–94.

Pope HG, Gruber AJ, Hudson JI, Cohane G, Huestis MA, Yurgelun-Todd D (2003). Early-onset cannabis use and cognitive deficits: what is the nature of the association? Drug Alcohol Depend. 69(3):303–10.

Schneider M (2012). The impact of pubertal exposure to cannabis on the brain: a focus on animal studies. In: Castle D, Murray R, D'Souza DC, editors. Marijuana and madness Cambridge: Cambridge University Press:82–90.

Solowij N, Jones KA, Rozman ME, Davis SM, Ciarrochi J, Heaven PC, et al. (2011). Verbal learning and memory in adolescent cannabis users, alcohol users and non-users. Psychopharmacology. 216(1):131–44.

Solowij N, Pesa N (2012). Cannabis and cognition: short and long-term effects. In: Castle D, Murray R, D'Souza DC, editors. Marijuana and madness, second edition. Cambridge: Cambridge University Press:91–102.

Sonon KE, Richardson GA, Cornelius JR, Kim KH, Day NL (2015). Prenatal marijuana exposure predicts marijuana use in young adulthood. Neurotoxicol Teratol. 47:10–5.

Tortoriello G, Morris CV, Alpar A, Fuzik J, Shirran SL, Calvigioni D, et al. (2014). Miswiring the brain: Delta9-tetrahydrocannabinol disrupts cortical development by inducing an SCG10/stathmin-2 degradation pathway. EMBO Journal. 33(7):668–85.

van der Pol P, Liebregts N, de Graaf R, Korf DJ, van den Brink W, van Laar M (2013). Predicting the transition from frequent cannabis use to cannabis dependence: a three-year prospective study. Drug Alcohol Depend. 133(2):352–9. doi:10.1016/j.drugalcdep.2013.06.009.

Verweij KJ, Zietsch BP, Lysnkey MT, Medland SE, Neale MC, Martin NG, et al. (2010). Genetic and environmental influences on cannabis use initiation and problematic use: a meta-analysis of twin studies. Addiction. 105(3):417–30.

Volkow ND, Baler RD, Compton WM, Weiss SR (2014a). Adverse health effects of marijuana use. NEJM. 370(23):2219–27.

Volkow ND, Wang GW, Telang F, Fowler JS, Alexoff D, Logan J, et al. (2014b). Decreased dopamine brain reactivity in marijuana abusers is associated with negative emotionality and addiction severity. Proc Natl Acad Sci U S A. 111(30):E3149–E3156.

Volkow N (2015). Cannabis and the central nervous system [background paper submitted to the WHO Scientific Meeting on Harms to Health due to Cannabis, Stockholm, 21–23 April 2015].

Yücel M, Solowij N, Respondek C, Whittle S, Fornito A, Pantelis C, et al. (2008). Regional brain abnormalities associated with long-term heavy cannabis use. Arch Gen Psychiatry. 65:694–701.

Yücel M, Lorenzetti V, Suo C, Zalesky A, Fornito A, Takagi MJ, et al. (2016). Hippocampal harms, protection and recovery following regular cannabis use. Transl Psychiatry. 6:e710.

Zalesky A, Solowij N, Yücel M, Lubman DI, Takagi M, Harding IH, et al. (2012). Effect of long-term cannabis use on axonal fibre connectivity. Brain. 135(Pt 7):2245–55.

Chapter 5

Asbridge M, Hayden JA, Cartwright JL (2012). Acute cannabis consumption and motor vehicle collision risk: systematic review of observational studies and meta-analysis. BMJ. 344:14–7.

Asbridge M, Mann R, Cusimano MD, Trayling C, Roerecke M, Tallon JM, et al. (2014). Cannabis and traffic collision risk: findings from a case-crossover study of injured drivers presenting to emergency departments. Int J Public Health. 59(2):395–404.

Berning A, Compton R, Wochinger K (2015). Results of the 2013–2014 National roadside survey of alcohol and drug use by drivers. Traffic Safety Facts Research Note, Report No. DOT HS 812 118. Washington (DC): National Highway Traffic Safety Administration.

Calabria B, Degenhardt L, Hall W, Lynskey M (2010b). Does cannabis use increase the risk of death? Systematic review of epidemiological evidence on adverse effects of cannabis use. Drug Alcohol Rev. 29:318–30.

Cherpitel CJ, Ye Y, Watters K, Brubacher JR, Strenstrom R (2012). Risk of injury from alcohol and drug use in the emergency department: a case-crossover study. Drug Alcohol Rev. 31(4):431–438.

Chesher G, Greeley J, Saunders J (1992). Tolerance to the effects of alcohol. In: Greeley J, Gladstone W, editors. The effects of alcohol on cognitive, psychomotor, and affective functioning. Kensington: National Drug and Alcohol Research Centre: 44–65.

Compton R, Berning A (2015). Drug and alcohol crash risk. Traffic Safety Facts Research Note, Report No. DOT HS 812 117. Washington (DC): National Highway Traffic Safety Administration.

Crean RD, Crane NA, Mason BJ (2011). An evidence based review of acute and long-term effects of cannabis use on executive cognitive functions. J Addict Med. 5(1):1–8.

Dines AM, Wood DM, Galicia M, Yates CM, Heyerdahl F, Hovda KE, et al. (2015). Presentations to the emergency department following cannabis use – a multi-centre case series from ten European countries. J Med Toxicol. 11(4):415-21.

Dubois S, Mullen N, Weaver B, Bédard M (2015). The combined effects of alcohol and cannabis on driving: impact on crash risk. Forensic Sci Int. 248: 94–100.

Elvik R (2015). Risk of road traffic injury associated with the use of drugs [background paper submitted to the WHO Technical Consultation on Drug Use and Road Safety, Geneva, Switzerland, 17-18 December 2014.

Fischer B, Imtiaz S, Rudzinski K, Rehm J (2015). Crude estimates of cannabis-attributable mortality and morbidity in Canada–implications for public health focused intervention priorities. J Public Health. doi:10.1093/pubmed/fdv005.

Gable RS (2004). Comparison of acute lethal toxicity of commonly abused psychoactive substances. Addiction. 99:686–96.

Gerberich S, Sidney S, Braun BL, Tekawa IS, Tolan KK, Quesenberry CP (2003). Marijuana use and injury events resulting in hospitalization. Ann epidemiol. 13(4):230–7.

Gmel G, Kuendig, H, Rehm J, Schreyer N, Daeppen JB (2009). Alcohol and cannabis use as risk factors for injury – a case-crossover analysis in a Swiss hospital emergency department. Biomed Central Public Health. 9:40.

Goldsmith RS, Targino MC, Fanciullo GJ, Martin DW, Hartenbaum NP, White JM, et al. (2015). Medical marijuana in the workplace: challenges and management options for occupational physicians. J Occup Environ Med. 57(5):518–25.

Hall W (2012). Driving while under the influence of cannabis (editorial). BMJ. 344:e595.

Hall WD, Solowij N, Lemon J (1994). The health and psychological consequences of cannabis use (vol. 25). Canberra: Australian Government Publishing Service.

Hartman RL, Huestis MA (2013). Cannabis effects on driving skills. Clin Chem. 59(3):478-92.

Hels T, Bernhoft IM, Lyckegaard A, Houwing S, Hagenzieker M, Legrand SA (2012). Risk of injury by driving with alcohol and other drugs. Revision 2.0 DRUID – Driving Under the Influence of Drugs, Alcohol and Medicines; sixth framework programme deliverable D2.3.5. Copenhagen: Danmarks Tekniske Universitet and partners for the European Commission.

Ilie G, Adlaf EM, Mann RE, Ialomiteanu A, Hamilton H, Rehm J, et al. (2015). Associations between a history of traumatic brain injuries and current cigarette smoking, substance use, and elevated psychological distress in a population sample of Canadian adults. J Neurotrauma. 32(14):1130–4.

Iversen L (2007). The science of marijuana, second edition. Oxford: Oxford University Press.

Iversen L (2012). How cannabis works in the human brain. In: Castle D, Murray R, D'Souza DC, editors. Marijuana and madness. Cambridge: Cambridge University Press:1–11.

Jouanjus E, Lapeyre-Mestre M, Micallef J (2014). Cannabis use: signal of increasing risk of serious cardiovascular disorders. J Am Heart Assoc. 3(2):e000638.

Lachenmeier DW, Rehm J (2015). Comparative risk assessment of alcohol, tobacco, cannabis and other illicit drugs using the margin of exposure approach. Sci Rep. 5:8126.

Laumon B, Gadegbeku B, Martin JL, Biecheler MB (2005). Cannabis intoxication and fatal road crashes in France: population based case-control study. BMJ. 331(7529):1371.

Leirer VO, Yesavage JA, Morrow DG (1991). Marijuana carry-over effects on aircraft pilot performance. Aviat Space Environ Med. 62(3):221–7.

Li MC, Brady JE, DiMaggio CJ, Lusardi AR, Tzong KY, Li G (2012). Marijuana use and motor vehicle crashes. Epidemiol Rev. 34(1):65–72.

Liakoni E, Dolder PC, Rentsch K, Liechti ME (2015). Acute health problems due to recreational drug use in patients presenting to an urban emergency department in Switzerland. Swiss Med Wkly. 145:w14166.

Macdonald S, Anglin-Bodrug K, Mann RE, Erickson P, Hathaway A, Chipman M, et al. (2003). Injury risk associated with cannabis and cocaine use. Drug Alcohol Depend. 72(2):99–115.

Mittleman MA, Lewis RA, Maclure M, Sherwood JB, Muller JE (2001). Triggering myocardial infarction by marijuana. Circulation. 103:2805–9.

Moskowitz H (1985). Marihuana and driving. Accid Anal Prev. 17(4):323–45.

Mura P, Kintz P, Ludes B, Gaulier JM, Marquet P, Martin-Dupont S, et al. (2003). Comparison of the prevalence of alcohol, cannabis and other drugs between 900 injured drivers and 900 control subjects: results of a French collaborative study. Forensic Sci Int. 133(1–2):79–85.

Pacher P, Kunos G (2013). Modulating the endocannabinoid system in human health and disease – successes and failures. FEBS J. 280(9):1918–43.

Phillips JA, Holland MG, Baldwin DD, Meuleveld LG, Mueller KL, Perkison B, et al. (2015). Marijuana in the workplace: guidance for occupational health professionals and employers: joint guidance statement of the American Association of Occupational Health Nurses and the American College of Occupational and Environmental Medicine. J Occup Environ Med. 57(4):459–75.

Ranganathan M, D'Souza DC (2006). The acute effects of cannabinoids on memory in humans: a review. Psychopharmacology. 188(4):425–44.

Robbe HWJ, O'Hanlon JF (1993). Marijuana and actual driving performance. Report No. DOT HS 808 078. Washington (DC): National Highway Traffic Safety Administration.

Robbe HW (1994). Influence of marijuana on driving. Maastricht: Institute for Human Psychopharmacology.

SAMHSA (2012). Drug Abuse Warning Network (DAWN) 2010: national estimates of drug related emergency department visits. HHS publication no. (SMA)12-4733, DAWN series D-38. Rockville (MD): Substance Abuse and Mental Health Services Administration.

SAMHSA (2013). Drug Abuse Warning Network (DAWN) 2011: national estimates of drug related emergency department visits. HHS publication no. (SMA)13-4760, DAWN Series D-39. Rockville (MD): Substance Abuse and Mental Health Services Administration.

Schmid K, Schönlebe J, Drexler H, Mueck-Weymann M (2010). The effects of cannabis on heart rate variability and well-being in young men. Pharmacopsychiatry. 43(4):147-50.

Smiley A (1999). Marijuana: on road and driving simulator studies. In: Kalant H, Corrigall W, Hall WD, et al., editors. The health effects of cannabis. Toronto: Centre for Addiction and Mental Health:171–91.

Smith DE (1968). Acute and chronic toxicity of marijuana. J Psychedelic Drugs. 2:37–47.

Tashkin DP (2015). Does marijuana pose risks for chronic airflow obstruction? Ann Am Thorac Soc. 12(2):235–6.

Thomas H (1993). Psychiatric symptoms in cannabis users. Brit J Psychiat. 163:141–9.

Weil A (1970). Adverse reactions to marijuana, classification, and suggested treatment. NEJM. 282:997–1000.

WHO (1997). Cannabis: a health perspective and research agenda. Geneva: World Health Organization:46.

Chapter 6

Advisory Council on the Misuse of Drugs (2008). Cannabis: classification and public health. London: Home Office.

Agrawal A, Lynskey MT (2009). Tobacco and cannabis co-occurrence: does route of administration matter? Drug Alcohol Depend. 99(1–3):240–7.

Agrawal A, Nurnberger JI Jr., Lynskey MT (2011). Cannabis involvement in individuals with bipolar disorder. Psychiatry Res. 185(3):459–61.

Ajdacic-Gross V, Lauber C, Warnke I, Haker H, Murray RM, Rössler W (2007). Changing incidence of psychotic disorders among the young in Zurich. Schizophren Res. 95(1–3):9–18.

Allsop DJ, Copeland J, Lintzeris N, Dunlop AJ, Montebello M, Sadler C, et al. (2012). Quantifying the clinical significance of cannabis withdrawal. PLoS One. 7(9):e44864.

Allsop DJ, Copeland J, Lintzeris N, Dunlop AJ, Montebello M, Sadler C, et al. (2014). Nabiximols as an agonist replacement therapy during cannabis withdrawal: a randomized clinical trial. JAMA Psychiatry. 71(3):281–91.

Andréasson S, Allebeck P (1990). Cannabis and mortality among young men: a longitudinal study of Swedish conscripts. Scand J Soc Med. 18:9–15.

Andréasson S, Allebeck P, Engström A, Rydeberg U (1987). Cannabis and schizophrenia: a longitudinal study of Swedish conscripts. Lancet. 2(8574):1483–6.

Anthony JC (2006). The epidemiology of cannabis dependence. In: Roffman RA, Stephens RS, editors. Cannabis dependence: its nature, consequences and treatment. Cambridge: Cambridge University Press:58–105.

Arendt M, Munk-Jørgensen P, Sher L, Wallenstein Jensen SO (2013). Mortality following treatment for cannabis use disorders: predictors and causes. J Subst Abuse Treat. 44(4):400-6.

Arseneault L, Cannon M, Poulton R, Murray R, Caspi A, Moffitt TE (2002). Cannabis use in adolescence and risk for adult psychosis: longitudinal prospective study. BMJ. 325(7374):1212–3.

Auer R, Vittinghoff E, Yaffe K, Künzi A, Kertesz SG, Levine DA, et al. (2016). Association between lifetime marijuana use and cognitive function in middle age: the Coronary Artery Risk Development in Young Adults (CARDIA) study. JAMA Intern Med. doi: 10.1001/jamainternalmed.2015.7841.

Bagge CL, Borges G (2015). The acute and chronic effects of cannabis on suicidal ideation, non fatal attempts, and death by suicide drugs [background paper submitted to the WHO Scientific Meeting on Harms to Health Due to Cannabis, Stockholm, 21–23 April 2015, available from the WHO Secretariat upon request].

Beautrais A, Joyce P, Mulder R (1999). Cannabis abuse and serious suicide attempts. Addiction. 94(8):1155–64.

Bergen SE, Gardner CO, Aggen SH, Kendler KS (2008). Socioeconomic status and social support following illicit drug use: causal pathways or common liability? Twin Res Hum Genet. 11(3):266–74.

Brook JS, Lee JY, Finch SJ, Seltzer N, Brook DW (2013). Adult work commitment, financial stability, and social environment as related to trajectories of marijuana use beginning in adolescence. Subst Abus. 34:298–305.

Borges G, Bagge CL, Orozco R (2016). A literature review and meta-analyses of cannabis use and suicidality. J Affect Disord. 195:63–74.

Borowsky IW, Ireland M, Resnick MD (2001). Adolescent suicide attempts: risks and protectors. Pediatrics. 107(3):485–93.

Bovasso GB (2001). Cannabis abuse as a risk factor for depressive symptoms. Am J Psych. 158(12):2033–7.

Boydell J, van Os J, Caspi A, Kennedy N, Giouroukou E, Fearon P, et al. (2006). Trends in cannabis use prior to first presentation with schizophrenia, in South-East London between 1965 and 1999. Psychol Med. 36(10):1441–6.

Budney AJ, Hughes JR (2006). The cannabis withdrawal syndrome. Curr Opin Psychiatry. 19:233–8.

CDC (2006). Web-based injury statistics query and reporting system (WISQARS™). Atlanta (GA): Centers for Disease Control and Prevention (http://www.cdc.gov/ncipc/wisqars, accessed 05 September 2015).

Clarke MC, Coughlan H, Harley M, Connor D, Power E, Lynch F, et al. (2014). The impact of adolescent cannabis use, mood disorder and lack of education on attempted suicide in young adulthood. World Psychiatry. 13(3):322–3.

Crane NA, Schuster RM, Fusar-Poli P, Gonzales, R (2013). Effects of cannabis on neurocognitive functioning: recent advances, neurodevelopmental influences, and sex differences. Neuropsychol Rev. 23(2):117–37.

Darke S, Duflou J, Torok M (2009). Drugs and violent death: comparative toxicology of homicide and non-substance toxicity suicide victims. Addiction. 104(6):1000–5.

Degenhardt L, Dierker L, Chiu WT, Medina-Mora, ME, Neumark Y, Sampson N, et al. (2010). Evaluating the drug use "gateway" theory using cross-national data: consistency and associations of the order of initiation of drug use among participants in the WHO World Mental Health Surveys. Drug Alcohol Depend. 108(1–2):84–97.

Degenhardt L, Hall WD (2012). Extent of illicit drug use and dependence, and their contribution to the global burden of disease. Lancet. 379(9810):55–70.

Di Forti M, Morgan C, Dazzan P, Pariante C, Mondelli V, Reis Marques T, et al. (2009). High-potency cannabis and the risk of psychosis. Brit J Psychiat. 195(6):488–91.

Di Forti M, Sallis H, Allegri F, Trotta A, Ferraro L, Stilo SA, et al. (2014). Daily use, especially of high-potency cannabis, drives the earlier onset of psychosis in cannabis users. Schizophr Bull. 40(6):1509–17.

Di Forti M, Marconi A, Carra E, Fraietta S, Trotta A, Bonomo M, et al. (2015). Proportion of patients in south London with first-episode psychosis attributable to use of high potency cannabis: a case-control study. Lancet Psychiatry. 2(3):233–8.

D'Souza DC, Perry E, Macdougall L, Ammerman Y, Cooper T, Wu YT, et al. (2004). The psychotomimetic effects of intravenous delta-9-tetrahydrocannabinol in healthy individuals: implications for psychosis. Neuropsychopharmacology. 29(8):1558–72.

D'Souza DC, Abi-Saab WM, Madonick S, Forselius-Bielen K, Doersch A, Braley G, et al (2005). Delta-9-tetrahydrocannabinol effects in schizophrenia: implications for cognition, psychosis, and addition. Biol Psychiatry. 57:594–608.

D'Souza DC, Sewell RA, Ranganathan M (2009). Cannabis and psychosis/schizophrenia: human studies. Eur Arch Psychiatry Clin Neurosci. 259(7):413–31.

Ellgren M, Spano SM, Hurd YL (2007) Adolescent cannabis exposure alters opiate intake and opioid limbic neuronal populations in adult rats. Neuropsychopharmacology. 32(3):607-15.

Ellgren M, Artmann A, Tkalych O, Gupta A, Hansen HS, Hansen SH, et al. (2008) Dynamic changes of the endogenous cannabinoid and opioid mesocorticolimbic systems during adolescence: THC effects. Eur Neuropsychopharmacol. 18(11):826–34.

Ellickson P, Bui K, Bell R, McGuigan KA (1998). Does early drug use increase the risk of dropping out of high school? J Drug Issues. 28(2):357–380.

EMCDDA (2011). Table TDI-105, part vii: all clients entering inpatient treatment by primary drug and age, 2009 or most recent year available: all cannabis inpatient clients by country and age. Statistical Bulletin 2011: Demand for Treatment (TDI). Lisbon: European Monitoring Centre for Drugs and Drug Addiction.

EMCDDA (2013). Drug treatment overview for Netherlands. Lisbon: European Monitoring Centre for Drugs and Drug Addiction (http://www.webcitation.org/6S4yjPY59, accessed 15 June 2015).

Feingold D, Weiser M, Rehm J, Lev-Ran S (2015). The association between cannabis use and mood disorders: a longitudinal study. J Affect Disord. 172:211–8.

Fergusson DM, Horwood L (1997). Early onset cannabis use and psychosocial adjustment in young adults. Addiction. 92(3):279–96.

Fergusson DM, Lynskey MT, Horwood LJ (1996). The short-term consequences of early onset cannabis use. J Abnorm Child Psych. 24(4):499–512.

Fergusson DM, Horwood LJ, Swain-Campbell NR (2003). Cannabis dependence and psychotic symptoms in young people. Psychol Med. 33:15–21.

Fergusson D, Boden J, Horwood L (2006). Cannabis use and other illicit drug use: testing the cannabis gateway hypothesis. Addiction. 101(4):556–69.

Fergusson D, Boden J, Horwood L (2008). The developmental antecedents of illicit drug use: evidence from a 25-year longitudinal study. Drug Alcohol Depend. 96(1–2):165–77.

Fergusson DM, Boden JM (2008) Cannabis use and later life outcomes. Addiction. 103(6):969–76.

Fergusson DM, Boden JM, Horwood LJ (2015) Psychosocial sequelae of cannabis use and implications for policy: findings from the Christchurch Health and Development Study. Soc Psychiatry Psychiatr Epidemiol. 50(9): 1317–26.

Fergusson D, Horwood L, Swain-Campbell N (2003). Cannabis dependence and psychotic symptoms in young people. Psychol Med. 33:15–21.

Fischer B, Imtiaz S, Rudzinski K, Rehm J (2015). Crude estimates of cannabis-attributable mortality and morbidity in Canada–implications for public health focused intervention priorities. J Pub Health. doi:10.1093/pubmed/fdv005 (Epub ahead of print).

Florez-Salamanca L, Secades-Villa R, Budney AJ, Garcia-Rodriguez O, Wang S, Blanco C (2013) Probability and predictors of cannabis use disorders relapse: results of the National Epidemiologic Survey on Alcohol and Related Conditions (NESARC). Drug Alcohol Depend. 132(1–2):127–33 (http://dx.doi.org/10.1016/j.drugalcdep, accessed 05 September 2015).

Gage SH, Zammit S, Hickman M (2013). Stronger evidence is needed before accepting that cannabis plays an important role in the aetiology of schizophrenia in the population. F1000 Medicine Reports. 5:2.

Giordano GN, Ohlsson H, Sundquist K, Sunquist J, Kendler K (2014). The association between cannabis abuse and subsequent schizophrenia: a Swedish national co-relative control study. Psychol Med. 45(2):407–414.

Goodman M, George T (2015). Is there a link between cannabis and mental illness? In: George T, Vaccarino F, editors. Substance abuse in Canada: the effects of cannabis use during adolescence. Ottawa: Canadian Centre on Substance Abuse:3247.

Grant I, Gonzalez R, Carey CL, Natarajan L, Wolfson T (2003). Non-acute (residual) neurocognitive effects of cannabis use: a meta-analytic study. J Int Neuropsychol Soc. 9(5):679–89.

Grant JD, Lynskey MT, Scherrer JF, Agrawal A, Heath AC, Bucholz KK (2010). A cotwin-control analysis of drug use and abuse/dependence risk associated with early-onset cannabis use. Addict Behav. 35:35–41.

Grant JD, Scherrer JF, Lynskey MT, Agrawal A, Duncan AE, Haber JR, et al. (2012). Associations of alcohol, nicotine, cannabis, and drug use/dependence with educational attainment: evidence from cotwin-control analyses. Alcohol Clin Exp Res. 36(8):1412–20.

Hall W, Degenhardt L, Teesson M (2009). Understanding comorbidity between substance use, anxiety and affective disorders: broadening the research base. Addict Behav. 34:526–30.

Hall WD, Lynskey M (2005). Is cannabis a gateway drug? Testing hypotheses about the relationship between cannabis use and the use of other illicit drugs. Drug Alcohol Rev. 24(1):39–48.

Hall W (2014). What has research over the past two decades revealed about the adverse health effects of recreational cannabis use? Soc Study Addict. 110:19–35.

Hall WD, Pacula RL (2010). Cannabis use and dependence: public health and public policy (reissue of first edition 2003). Cambridge: Cambridge University Press.

Hall WD, Solowij N, Lemon J (1994). The health and psychological consequences of cannabis use (vol. 25). Canberra: Australian Government Publishing Service.

Haney M, Evins AE (2016). Does cannabis cause, exacerbate or ameliorate psychiatric disorders? An oversimplified debate discussed. Neuropsychopharmacology. 41(2):393–401.

Hasin, D, Tulshi D, Kerridge B, Goldstein R, Chou P, Zhang H, et al. (2015) Prevalence of marijuana use disorders in the United States between 2001-2002 and 2012-2013. JAMA Psychiatry. 72(12):1235–42. doi:10.1001/jamapsychiatry.2015.1858.

Henquet C, Krabbendam L, Spauwen J, Kaplan C, Lieb R, Wittchen HW, et al. (2004). Prospective cohort study of cannabis use, predisposition for psychosis, and psychotic symptoms in young people. British Medical Journal. 330(7481):11.

Henquet C, Krabbendam L, de Graaf R, ten Have M, van Os J (2006). Cannabis use and expression of mania in the general population. Journal of Affective Disorders. 95(1-3):103-110.

Hibell B, Guttormsson U, Ahlström S, Balakireva O, Bjarnason T, Kokkevi A (2012). The 2011 ESPAD report: substance use among students in 36 European countries (http://www.espad.org/Uploads/ESPAD_reports/2011). Stockholm: the Swedish Council for Information on Alcohol and Other Drugs (CAN).

Hickman M, Vickerman P, Macleod J, Kirkbride J, Jones PB (2007). Cannabis and schizophrenia: model projections of the impact of the rise in cannabis use on historical and future trends in schizophrenia in England and Wales. Addiction. 102(4):597–606.

Horwood LJ, Fergusson DM, Hayatbakhsh MR, Najman JM, Coffey C, Patton GC, et al. (2010). Cannabis use and educational achievement: findings from three Australasian cohort studies. Drug Alcohol Depend. 110(3):247–53.

Horwood LJ, Fergusson DM, Coffey C, Patton GC, Tait R, Smart D, et al. (2012). Cannabis and depression: an integrative data analysis of four Australasian cohorts. Drug Alcohol Depend. 126(3):369–78.

Johnston LD, O'Malley PM, Bachman JG, Schulenberg JE (2010). Marijuana use is rising; ecstasy use is beginning to rise; and alcohol use is declining among U.S. teens. Press release. Ann Arbor (MI): University of Michigan News Service (http://www.monitoringthefuture.org/pressreleases/10drugpr_complete.pdf, accessed 11 February 2016).

Jorquera N, Alvarado R, Libuy N, de Angel V (2015). Association between unmet needs and clinical status in patients with first episode of schizophrenia in Chile. Front Psychiatry. 6(57). doi: 10.3389/fpsyt.2015.00057.

Juon HS, Ensminger ME (1997). Childhood, adolescent, and young adult predictors of suicidal behaviors: a prospective study of African Americans. J Child Psychol. 38(5):553–63.

Kandel D (2002). Stages and pathways of drug involvement: examining the gateway hypothesis. New York: Cambridge University Press.

Kung HC, Pearson JL, Liu X. (2003). Risk factors for male and female suicide decedents ages 15-64 in the United States. Results from the 1993 National Mortality Followback Survey. Soc Psychiatry Psychiatr Epidemiol. 38(8):419–26.

Kung HC, Pearson JL, Wei R (2005). Substance use, firearm availability, depressive symptoms, and mental health service utilization among white and African American suicide decedents aged 15 to 64 years. Ann epidemiol. 15(8):614–21.

Lai H, Sitharthan T (2012). Exploration of the comorbidity of cannabis use disorders and mental health disorders among inpatients presenting to all hospitals in New South Wales, Australia. Am J Drug Alcohol Abuse. 38(6):567–74.

Lessem J, Hopfer CJ, Haberstick BC, Timberlake D, Ehringer MA, Smolen A, et al. (2006). Relationship between adolescent marijuana use and young adult illicit drug use. Behav Genet. 36(4):498–506.

Lev-Ran S, Le Foll B, McKenzie K, George TP, Rehm J (2013). Bipolar disorder and co-occurring cannabis use disorders: characteristics, co-morbidities and clinical correlates. Psychiatry Res. 209(3):459–65.

Lorenzetti V, Lubman DI, Fornito A, Whittle S, Takagi MJ, Solowij N, et al. (2013). The impact of regular cannabis use on the human brain: a review of structural neuroimaging studies. In: Miller PM, editor. Biological research on addiction. San Diego (CA): Academic Press: 711–28.

Lichtman A, Martin B (2005). Cannabinoid tolerance and dependence. Handbook of Experimental Pharmacology. 168:691–717.

Lynskey M, Hall W (2000). The effects of adolescent cannabis use on educational attainment: a review. Addiction. 95(11):1621–30.

Lynskey MT, Heath AC, Bucholz KK, Slutske WS, Madden PAF, Nelson EC, et al. (2003). Escalation of drug use in early-onset cannabis users vs co-twin controls. JAMA. 289(4):427-33.

Lynskey MT, Vink JM, Boomsma DI (2006). Early onset cannabis use and progression to other drug use in a sample of Dutch twins. Behav Genet. 36(2):195–200.

Manrique-Garcia E, Zamit S, Dalman C, Hemmingsson T, Allebeck P (2012). Cannabis use and depression: a longitudinal study of a national cohort of Swedish conscripts. BMC Psychiatry. 12(112). doi:10.1186/1471-244X-12-112.

McGee R, Williams S, Nada-Raja S (2005). Is cigarette smoking associated with suicidal ideation among young people? Am J Psych. 162(3):619–20.

McGrath J, Welham J, Scott J, Varghese D, Degenhardt L, Hayatbakhsh MR, et al. (2010). Association between cannabis use and psychosis-related outcomes using sibling pair analysis in a cohort of young adults. Arch Gen Psychiatry. 67(5):440–47.

Meier MH, Caspi A, Ambler A, Harrington H, Houts R, Keefe RS, et al. (2012). Persistent cannabis users show neuropsychological decline from childhood to midlife. Proc Natl Acad Sci U S A. 109(40):E2657–64.

Moffitt TE, Meier MH, Caspi A, Poulton R (2013). Reply to Rogeberg & Daly: no evidence that socioeconomic status or personality differences confound the association between cannabis use and IQ decline. Proc Natl Acad Sci U S A. 110(11):E980–2.

Moore T, Zammit S, Lingford-Hughes A, Barnes TRE, Jones PB, Burke M, et al. (2007). Cannabis use and risk of psychotic or affective mental health outcomes: a systematic review. Lancet. 370(9584):319–28.

Morral A, McCaffrey D, Paddock S (2002). Reassessing the marijuana gateway effect. Addiction. 97(12):1493–504.

Morrison PD, Zois V, Mckeown DA, Lee TD, Holt DW, Powell JF, et al. (2009). The acute effects of synthetic intravenous delta9-tetrahydrocannabinol on psychosis, mood and cognitive functioning. Psychol Med. 39(10):1607–16.

Moussavi S, Chatterji S, Verdes E, Tandon A, Patel V, Ustun B (2007). Depression, chornic diseases, and decrements in health: results from the World Health Surveys. Lancet. 370(9590):851–8.

Murray RM, Paparelli A, Morrison PD, Marconi A, Di Forti M (2013). What can we learn about schizophrenia from studying the human model, drug-induced psychosis? Am J Med Genet B Neuropsychiatr Genet. 162B:661–70.

Myles H, Myles N, Large M (2015). Cananbis use in first episode psychosis: meta-analysis of prevalence, and the time course of initiation and continued use. Australasian and NZ J of Psychiatry. doi: 10.1177/0004867415599846 (Epub ahead of print).

Newcomb MD, Scheier LM, Bentler PM (1993). Effects of adolescent drug use on adult mental health: a prospective study of a community sample. Exp Clin Psychopharm. 1(1–4):215–41.

Newcomb MD, Vargas-Carmona J, Galaif ER (1999). Drug problems and psychological distress among a community sample of adults: predictors, consequences, or confound? J Community Psychol. 27(4):405–29.

Patton GC, Coffey C, Carlin JB, Sawyer SM, Lynskey M (2005). Reverse gateways? Frequent cannabis use as a predictor of tobacco initiation and nicotine dependence. Addiction. 100(10):1518–25.

Pedersen W (2008). Does cannabis use lead to depression and suicidal behaviours? A population-based longitudinal study. Acta Psychiatrica Scandinavica. 118(5):395–403.

Petronis KR, Samuels JF, Moscicki EK, Anthony JC (1990). An epidemiologic investigation of potential risk factors for suicide attempts. Soc Psychiatry Psychiatr Epidemiol. 25(4):193-9.

Palacio C, Garcia J, Diago J, Zapata C, Lopez G, Ortiz J, et al. (2007) Identification of suicide risk factors in Medellin Colombia: a case-control study of psychological autopsy in a developing country. Arch Suicide Res. 11(3):297–308.

Power RA, Verweij KJH, Zuhair M, Montgomery GW, Henders AK, Heath AC, et al. (2014). Genetic predisposition to schizophrenia associated with increased use of cannabis. Molecular Psychiatry. 19(11):1201–4.

Price C, Hemmingsson T, Lewis G, Zammit S, Allebeck P (2009). Cannabis and suicide: longitudinal study. Brit J Psychiat. 195(6):492–7.

Roxburgh A, Hall WD, Degenhardt L, McLaren J, Black E, Copeland J, et al. (2010). The epidemiology of cannabis use and cannabis-related harm in Australia 1993–2007. Addiction. 105(6):1071–9.

Rogeberg O (2013). Correlations between cannabis use and IQ change in the Dunedin cohort are consistent with confounding from socioeconomic status. Proc Natl Acad Sci USA. 110(11):4251–4.

Schizophrenia Working Group of the Psychiatric Genomics Consortium (2014). Biological insights from 108 schizophrenia associated genetic loci. Nature. 511:421–427.

Schreiner A, Dunne ME (2012). Residual effects of cannabis use on neurocognitive performance after prolonged abstinence: a meta-analysis. Exp Clin Psychopharmacol. 20:420–9.

Sheehan CM, Rogers RJ, Williams GW, Boardman JD (2013). Gender differences in the presence of drugs in violent deaths. Addiction. 108(3):547–55.

Shields LB, Hunsaker DM, Hunsaker JC III, Ward MK (2006). Toxicologic findings in suicide: a 10-year retrospective review of Kentucky medical examiner cases. Am J Forensic Med Pathol 27(2):106–12.

Silberberg C, Castle D, Koethe D (2012). Cannabis, cannabinoids, and bipolar disorder. In: Castle D, Murray R, D'Souza DC, editors. Marijuana and madness, second edition. New York (NY): Cambridge University Press:129–36.

Silins E, Horwood LJ, Patton GC, Fergusson DM, Olsson CA, Hutchinson DM, et al. (2014). Young adult sequelae of adolescent cannabis use: an integrative analysis. Lancet Psychiatry. 1(4):286–93.

Solowij N (2002). Cannabis and cognitive functioning. In: Onaivi ES, editor. Biology of marijuana: from gene to behaviour. London: Taylor & Francis.

Solowij N, Battisti R (2008). The chronic effects of cannabis on memory in humans: a review. Curr Drug Abuse Rev. 1(1):81–98.

Solowij N, Jones KA, Rozman ME, Davis SM, Ciarrochi J, Heaven PCL, et al. (2011). Verbal learning and memory in adolescent cannabis users, alcohol users and non-users. Psychopharmacology. 216(1):131–44.

Solowij N, Pesa N (2012). Cannabis and cognition: short and long term effects. In: Castle D, Murray R, D'Souza DC, editors. Marijuana and madness, second edition. New York (NY): Cambridge University Press:91–102.

Stefanis NC, Dragovic M, Power BD, Jablensky A, Castle D, Morgan VA (2014). The effect of drug use on the age at onset of psychotic disorders in an Australian cohort. Schizophr Res. 156: 211–6.

Swift W, Hall W, Teesson, M (2001) Cannabis use and dependence among Australian adults: results from the National Survey of Mental Health and Well-being. Addiction. 96: 737–48.

Swift W, Coffey C, Degenhardt L, Carlin JB, Romaniuk H, Patton GC (2012). Cannabis and progression to other substance use in young adults: findings from a 13-year prospective population-based study. J Epidemiol Commun H 66(7):e26.

Therapeutic Goods Administration (2013). Australian public assessment report for Nabiximols: proprietary product name: Sativex. Sponsor: Novartis Pharmaceuticals Australia Pty Limited. Canberra: Commonwealth of Australia.

Tomasiewicz HC, Jacobs MM, Wilkinson MB, Wilson SP, Nestler EJ, Hurd YL (2012). Proenkephalin mediates the enduring effects of adolescent cannabis exposure associated with adult opiate vulnerability. Biol Psychiatry. 72(10):803–10.

Ustün TB, Ayuso-Mateos JL, Chatterji S, Mathers C, Murray CJ (2004). Global burden of depressive disorders in the year 2000. Brit J Psychiat. 184:386–92.

van der Pol P, Liebregts N, de Graaf R, Korf DJ, van den Brink W, van Laar M (2013). Predicting the transition from frequent cannabis use to cannabis dependence: a three-year prospective study. Drug Alcohol Depend. 133(2):352–9. doi:10.1016/j.drugalcdep.2013.06.009.

van Os J, Bak M, Hanssen M, Bijl RV, De Graaf R, Verdoux H. (2002). Cannabis use and psychosis: a longitudinal population-based study. Am J Epidemiol. 156(4):319–27.

van Ours JC, Williams J, Fergusson D, Horwood LJ (2013). Cannabis use and suicidal ideation. J Health Econ. 32(3):524–37.

Verweij KJH, Huizink AC, Agrawal A, Martin NG, Lynskey MT (2013). Is the relationship between early-onset cannabis use and educational attainment causal or due to common liability? Drug Alcohol Depend. 133(2):580–6. doi:10.1016/j.drugalcdep.2013.07.034.

Wagner F, Anthony J (2002). Into the world of illegal drug use: Exposure opportunity and other mechanisms linking the use of alcohol, tobacco, marijuana, and cocaine. Am J Epidemiol. 155(10):918–25.

Wichstrom L (2000). Predictors of adolescent suicide attempts: a nationally representative longitudinal study of Norwegian adolescents. J Acad Child Psy. 39(5):603–10.

WHO (1992). The ICD-10 classification of mental and behavioural disorders: clinical descriptions and diagnostic guidelines. Geneva: World Health Organization.

Wilcox HC, Anthony JC (2004). The development of suicide ideation and attempts: an epidemiologic study of first graders followed into young adulthood. Drug Alcohol Depend. 76 Suppl:S53–67.

Yücel M, Solowij N, Respondek C, Whittle S, Fornito A, Pantellis C, et al. (2008). Regional brain abnormalities associated with long-term heavy cannabis use. Arch Gen Psychiatry. 65:694–701.

Zammit S, Allebeck P, Andreasson S, Lundberg I, Lewis G (2002). Self-reported cannabis use as a risk factor for schizophrenia in Swedish conscripts of 1969: historical cohort study. BMJ. 325(7374):1199–201.

Zhang X, Wu LT (2014). Suicidal ideation and substance use among adolescents and young adults: a bidirectional relation? Drug Alcohol Depend. 142:63–73.

Chapter 7

Aldington S, Williams M, Nowitz M, Weatherall M, Pritchard A, Mcnaughton A, et al. (2007). Effects of cannabis on pulmonary structure, function and symptoms. Thorax. 62(12):1058–63.

Aldington S, Harwood M, Cox B, Weatherall M, Beckert L, Hansell A, et al. (2008a). Cannabis use and cancer of the head and neck: case-control study. JAMA Otolaryngol Head Neck Surg. 138(3):374–80.

Aldington S, Harwood M, Cox B, Weatherall M, Beckert L, Hansell A, et al. (2008b). Cannabis use and risk of lung cancer: a case-control study. Eur Respir J. 31(2):280–6.

Aronow WS, Cassidy J (1974). Effect of marijuana and placebo-marijuana smoking on Angina Pectoris. NEJM. 291:65–7.

Arora S, Goyal H, Aggarwal P, Kukar A (2012). ST-segment elevation myocardial infarction in a 37-year-old man with normal coronaries – it is not always cocaine! Am J Emerg Med 30(9):2091.e3–5.

Bailly C, Merceron O, Hammoudi N, Dorent R, Michel PL (2010). Cannabis induced acute coronary syndrome in a young female. Int J Cardiol. 143(1):e4–6.

Baldwin GC, Tashkin DP, Buckley DM, Park AN, Dubinett SM, Roth MD (1997) Marijuana and cocaine impair alveolar macrophage function and cytokine production. Am J Respir Crit Care Med. 156(5):1606–13.

Barber PA, Pridmore HM, Krishnamurthy V, Roberts S, Spriggs DA, Carter KN, et al. (2013). Cannabis, ischemic stroke, and transient ischemic attack: a case-control study. Stroke, 44(8):2327–9.

Basnet S, Mander G, Nicolas R (2009). Coronary vasposasm in an adolescent resulting from marijuana use. Pediatr Cardiol. 30(4):543–5.

Benson-Leung ME, Leung LY, Kumar S (2014). Synthetic cannabis and acute ischemic stroke. J Stroke Cerebrovasc Dis. 23(5):1239–41.

Berthiller J, Straif K, Boniol M, Voirin N, Benhaïm-Luzon V, Ayoub WB, et al. (2008). Cannabis smoking and risk of lung cancer in men: a pooled analysis of three studies in Maghreb. J Thorac Oncol. 3(12):1398–403.

Bloom JW, Kaltenborn WT, Paoletti P, Camilli A, Lebowitz MD (1987). Respiratory effects of non-tobacco cigarettes. BMJ. 295:1516–8.

Callaghan RC, Allebeck P, Sidorchuk A (2013). Marijuana use and risk of lung cancer: a 40-year cohort study. Cancer Causes Control. 24(10):1811–20.

Canga Y, Osmonov D, Karatas MB, Durmus G, Ilhan E, Kirbas V (2011). Cannabis: a rare trigger of premature myocardial infarction. Anadolu Kardiyol Derg [The Anatolian Journal of Cardiology]. 11(3):272–4.

Casier I, Vanduynhoven P, Haine S, Vrints C, Jorens PG (2013). Is recent cannabis use associated with acute coronary syndromes? Acta Cardiol. 69(2):131–6.

Chesher G, Hall W (1999). Effects of cannabis on the cardiovascular and gastrointestinal systems. In: Kalant H, Corrigall W, Hall WD, et al., editors. The health effects of cannabis. Toronto: Centre for Addiction and Mental Health:435–58.

Daling JR, Doody DR, Sun X, Trabert BL, Weiss NS, Chen C, et al. (2009). Association of marijuana use and the incidence of testicular germ cell tumors. Cancer. 115(6):1215–23.

Desbois AC, Cacoub P (2013). Cannabis-associated arterial disease. Ann Vasc Surg. 27(7):996–1005.

Deharo P, Massoure PL, Fourcade L (2013). Exercise-induced acute coronary syndrome in a 24-year-old man with massive cannabis consumption. Acta Cardiol. 68(4):425–8.

Duchene C, Olindo S, Chausson N, Jeannin S, Cohen-Tenoudji P, Smadja D (2010). Cannabis-induced cerebral and myocardial infarction in a young woman. Rev Neurol. 166:438–42.

Feng BJ, Ben-Ayoub W, Dahmoul S, Ayad M, Maachi F, Bedadra W, et al. (2009). Cannabis, tobacco and domestic fumes intake are associated with nasopharyngeal carcinoma in North Africa. Br J Cancer. 101(7):1207–12.

Fligiel SE, Roth MD, Kleerup EC, Barsky SH, Simmons MS, Tashkin DP (1997). Tracheobronchial histopathology in habitual smokers of cocaine, marijuana, and/or tobacco. Chest. 112(2):319–26.

Freeman MJ, Rose DZ, Myers MA, Gooch CL, Bozeman AC, Burgin WS (2013). Ischemic stroke after use of the synthetic marijuana "spice". Neurology. 81(24):2090–3.

Frost L, Mostofsky E, Rosenbloom JI, Mukamal KJ, Mittleman MA (2013). Marijuana use and long-term mortality among survivors of acute myocardial infarction. Am Heart J. 165(2):170–5.

Gillison ML, D'Souza G, Westra W, Sugar E, Xiao W, Begum S, et al. (2008). Distinct risk factor profiles for human papillomavirus type 16-positive and human papillomavirus type 16-negative head and neck cancers. J Natl Cancer Inst. 100(6):407–20.

Gottschalk L, Aronow W, Prakash R (1977). Effect of marijuana and placebo-marijuana smoking on psychological state and on psychophysiological and cardiovascular functioning in angina patients. Biol Psychiatry. 12(2):255–66.

Grufferman S, Schwartz AG, Ruyman FB, Maurer HM (1993). Parents' use of cocaine and marijuana and increased risk of rhabdomyosarcoma in their children. Cancer Causes Control. 4(3):217–24.

Gurney J, Young J, Roffers S, Smith MA, Bunin C (2000). Soft tissue sarcomas. In: Reis L, Eisner M, Kosary C, et al., editors. SEER Cancer Statistics Review, 1973–1997. Bethesda: National Cancer Institute:11–123.

Gurney J, Shaw C, Stanley J, Signal V, Sarfati D (2015) Cannabis exposure and risk of testicular cancer: a systematic review and meta-analysis. BMC Cancer. 15:897. doi: 10.1186/s12885-015-1905-6.

Hackam DG (2015). Cannabis and stroke. Stroke. 46:852–6.

Hall W, Macphee D (2002). Cannabis use and cancer. Addiction. 97:243–47.

Hancox RJ, Poulton R, Ely M, Welch D, Taylor DR, McLachlan CR, et al. (2010). Effects of cannabis on lung function: a population-based cohort study. Eur Respir J. 35(1):42–7.

Hancox RJ, Shin HH, Gray AR, Poulton R, Searson MR (2015). Effects of quitting cannabis on respiratory symptoms. Eur Respir J. 46(1):80–7.

Hashibe M, Morgenstern H, Cui Y, Tashkin DP, Zhang ZF, Cozen W, et al. (2006). Marijuana use and the risk of lung and upper aerodigestive tract cancers: results of a population-based case-control study. Cancer Epidemiol Biomarkers Prev. 15(10):1829–34.

Hashibe M, Straif K, Tashkin DP, Morgenstern H, Greenland S, Zhang ZF (2005). Epidemiologic review of marijuana use and cancer risk. Alcohol. 35(3):265–75.

Hii S, Tam JDC, Thompson BR, Naughton MT (2008). Bullous lung disease due to marijuana. Respirology. 13:122–7.

Hodcroft CJ, Rossiter MC, Buch AN (2014). Cannabis-associated myocardial infarction in a young man with normal coronary arteries. J Emerg Med. 47(3):277–81.

Johnson MK, Smith RP, Morrison D, Laszlo G, White RJ (2000). Large lung bullae in marijuana smokers. Thorax. 55:340–2.

Jones RT (2002). Cardiovascular system effects of marijuana. J Clin Pharmacol. 42(11): 58S–63S.

Jouanjus E, Lapeyre-Mestre M, Micallef J (2014). Cannabis use: signal of increasing risk of serious cardiovascular disorders. J Am Heart Assoc. 3(2):e000638.

Jouanjus E, Leymarie F, Tubery M, Lapeyre-mestre M (2011). Cannabis-related hospitalizations: unexpected serious events identified through hospital databases. Brit J Clin Pharmaco. 71(5):758–65.

Jouanjus E, Pourcel L, Saivin S, Molinier L, Lapeyre-mestre M (2012). Use of multiple sources and capture-recapture method to estimate the frequency of hospitalizations related to drug abuse. Pharmacoepidemiol Drug Saf. 21(7):733–41.

Joy JE, Watson SJ, Benson JA, editors. Marijuana and medicine: assessing the science base. Washington (DC): The National Academies Press (http://iom.edu/Reports/2003/Marijuana-and-Medicine-Assessing-the-Science-Base.aspx, accessed 05 September 2015).

Kagen SL, Kurup VP, Sohnle PC, Fink JN (1983). Marijuana smoking and fungal sensitization. J Allergy Clin Immunol. 71:389–93.

Karabulut A, Cakmak M (2010). ST segment elevation myocardial infarction due to slow coronary flow occurring after cannabis consumption. Kardiol Pol [Polish Heart Journal]. 68(11):1266–8.

Kempker JA, Honig EG, Martin GS (2015). The effects of marijuana exposure on expiratory airflow. A study of adults who participated in the U.S. National Health and Nutrition Examination Study. Ann Am Thorac Soc. 12(2):135–141.

Kocabay G, Yildiz M, Duran NE, Ozkan M (2009). Acute inferior myocardial infarction due to cannabis smoking in a young man. J Cardiovasc Med. 10:669–70.

Kuijten RR, Bunin GR, Nass CC, Meadows AT (1992). Parental occupation and childhood astrocytoma: results of a case control study. Cancer Res. 52(4):782–6.

Lacson JCA, Carroll JD, Tuazon E, Castelao EJ, Bernstein L, Cortessis VK (2012). Population-based case-control study of recreational drug use and testis cancer risk confirms an association between marijuana use and nonseminoma risk. Cancer. 118(21):5374–83.

Leuchtenberger C (1983). Effects of marihuana (cannabis) smoke on cellular biochemistry of in vitro test systems. In: Fehr K, Kalant H, editors Cannabis and health hazards. Toronto: Addiction Research Foundation.

Liang C, Mcclean MD, Marsit C, Christensen B, Peters E, Nelson H, et al. (2009). A population-based case-control study of marijuana use and head and neck squamous cell carcinoma. Cancer Prev Res. 2(8):759–68.

Llewellyn CD, Johnson NW, Warnakulasuriya KA (2004). Risk factors for oral cancer in newly diagnosed patients aged 45 years and younger: a case-control study in Southern England. J Oral Pathol Med. 33(9):525–32.

Llewellyn CD, Linklater K, Bell J, Johnson NW, Warnakulasuriya S (2004). An analysis of risk factors for oral cancer in young people: a case-control study. Oral Oncol. 40(3):304–13.

MacPhee D (1999). Effects of marijuana on cell nuclei: a review of the literature relating to the genotoxicity of cannabis. In: Kalant H, Corrigall W, Hall WD, et al., editors. The health effects of cannabis. Toronto: Centre for Addiction and Mental Health:435–58.

Marks MA, Chaturvedi AK, Kelsey K, Straif K, Berthiller J, Schwartz SM, et al. (2014). Association of marijuana smoking with oropharyngeal and oral tongue cancers: pooled analysis from the INHANCE consortium. Cancer Epidemiol Biomarkers Prev. 23(1):160–71.

Marselos M, Karamanakos P (1999). Mutagenicity, developmental toxicity and carcinogeneity of cannabis. Addict Biol. 4(1):5–12.

Mehra R, Serebriiskii IG, Dunbrack RL, Robinson MK, Burtness B, Golemis EA (2006). The association between marijuana smoking and lung cancer: a systematic review. Arch Intern Med. 166(13):1359–67.

Mittleman MA, Lewis RA, Maclure M, Sherwood JB, Muller JE (2001). Triggering myocardial infarction by marijuana. Circulation. 103:2805–9.

Mittleman MA, Mintzer D, Maclure M, Tofler GH, Sherwood JB, Muller JE (1999). Triggering myocardial infarction by cocaine. Circulation. 99(21):2737–41.

Montecucco F, Di Marzo V (2012). At the heart of the matter: the endocannabinoid system in cardiovascular function and dysfunction. Trends Pharmacol Sci. 33(6):331–40.

Moore BA, Augustson EM, Moser RP, Budney AJ (2005). Respiratory effects of marijuana and tobacco use in a U.S. sample. J Gen Intern Med. 20(1):33–7.

Mukamal KJ, Maclure M, Muller JE, Mittleman MA (2008). An exploratory prospective study of marijuana use and mortality following acute myocardial infarction. Am Heart J. 155(3):465–70.

Phan TD, Lau KKP, Li X (2005). Lung bullae and pulmonary fibrosis associated with marijuana smoking. Australas Radiol. 49:411–4.

Pletcher MJ, Vittinghoff E, Kalhan R, Richman J, Safford M, Sidney S, et al. (2012). Association between marijuana exposure and pulmonary function over 20 years. JAMA. 307(2):173–81.

Pratap B, Korniyenko A (2012). Toxic effects of marijuana on the cardiovascular system. Cardiovasc Toxicol. 12:143–8.

Reis L, Eisner M, Kosary C, Hankey B, Miller B, Clegg L, et al., editors (2000). SEER cancer statistics review, 1973–1997. Bethesda: National Cancer Institute.

Renard D, Taieb G, Gras-Combe G, Labauge P (2012). Cannabis-related myocardial infarction and cardioembolic stroke. J Stroke Cerebrovasc Dis. 21:82–3.

Robinson L, Buckley J, Daigle A, Wells R, Benjamin D, Arthur D, et al. (1989). Maternal drug use and the risk of childhood nonlymphoblastic leukemia among offspring: an epidemiologic investigation implicating marijuana. Cancer. 63:1904–11.

Rosenblatt KA, Daling JR, Chen C, Sherman KJ, Schwarts SM (2004). Marijuana use and risk of oral squamous cell carcinoma. Cancer Res. 64(11):4049–54.

Roth MD, Arora A, Barsky SH, Kleerup EC, Simmons M, Tashkin DP. (1998). Airway inflammation in young marijuana and tobacco smokers. Am J Respir Crit Care Med. 157(3 Part 1):928–37.

Sherrill DL, Krzyzanowski M, Bloom JW, Lebowitz MD (1991). Respiratory effects of non-tobacco cigarettes: a longitudinal study in general population. Int J Epidemiol. 20:132–7.

Sidney S, Quesenberry CP, Friedman GD, Tekawa IS (1997). Marijuana use and cancer incidence (California, United States). Cancer Causes Control. 8(5):722–8.

Sidney S (2002). Cardiovascular consequences of marijuana use. J Clin Pharmacol. 42(11 Suppl):64S–70S.

Smith MA, Gloekler-Reiss LA, Gurney J, Ross J (2000). Leukemia. In: Ries L, Smith MA, Gurney JG, et al., editors. SEER Cancer Statistics Review, 1973–1997. Bethesda: National Cancer Institute:17–34.

Takematsu M, Hoffman RS, Nelson LS, Schechter JM, Moran JH, Wiener SW (2014). A case of acute cerebral ischemia following inhalation of a synthetic cannabinoid. Clin Toxicol. 52(9):973.

Tan C, Hatam N, Treasure T (2006). Bullous disease of the lung and cannabis smoking: insufficient evidence for a causative link. J R Soc Med. 99(2):77–80.

Tan WC, Lo C, Jong A, Xing L, Fitzgerald MJ, Vollmer WM, et al. (2009). Marijuana and chronic obstructive lung disease: a population-based study. Can Med Assoc J. 180(8):814–20.

Tashkin DP (2015). Does marijuana pose risks for chronic airflow obstruction? Ann Am Thorac Soc. 12(2):235–36.

Tashkin DP, Calvarese BM, Simmons MS, Shapiro BJ (1980). Respiratory status of seventy-four habitual marijuana smokers. Chest. 78(5):699–706.

Tashkin DP, Coulson AH, Clark VA, Simmons M, Bourque LB, Duann S, et al. (1987). Respiratory symptoms and lung function in habitual heavy smokers of marijuana alone, smokers of marijuana and tobacco, smokers of tobacco alone, and non-smokers. Am Rev Respir Dis. 135:209–16.

Tashkin DP, Simmons MS, Sherrill DL, Coulson AH (1997). Heavy habitual marijuana smoking does not cause an accelerated decline in FEV1 with age. Am J Respir Crit Care Med. 155(1):141–8.

Tashkin DP, Simmons MS, Tseng CH (2012). Impact of changes in regular use of marijuana and/or tobacco on chronic bronchitis. COPD. 9(4):367–74.

Taylor DR, Poulton R, Moffitt TE, Ramankutty P, Sears MR (2000). The respiratory effects of cannabis dependence in young adults. Addiction. 95:1669–77.

Trabert B, Sigurdson AJ, Sweeney AM, Strom SS, Mcglynn KA (2011). Marijuana use and testicular germ cell tumors. Cancer. 117(4):848–53.

Ungerleider JT, Andrysiak T, Tashkin DP, Gale RP (1982). Contamination of marihuana cigarettes with pathogenic bacteria -- possible source of infection in cancer patients. Cancer Treat Rep. 66:589–91.

Van Hoozen BE, Cross CE (1997). Marijuana. Respiratory tract effects. Clin Rev Allergy Immunol. 15(3):243–69.

Wang X, Derakhshandeh R, Narayan S, Luu E, Le S, Danforth OM, et al. (2014). Brief exposure to marijuana secondhand smoke impairs vascular endothelial function [abstract]. Circulation. 130:A19538.

Wolff V, Armspach JP, Lauer V, Rouyer O, Bataillard M, Marescaux C, et al. (2013). Cannabis-related stroke: myth or reality? Stroke. 44(2):558–63.

Wolff V, Lauer V, Rouyer O, Sellal F, Meyer N, Raul J, et al. (2011). Cannabis use, ischemic stroke, and multifocal intracranial vasoconstriction: a prospective study in 48 consecutive young patients. Stroke. 42(6):1778–80.

Wolff V, Zinchenko I, Quenardelle V, Rouyer O, Geny B (2015). Characteristics and prognosis of ischemic stroke in young cannabis users compared with non-cannabis users. J Am Coll Cardiol. 66(18):2052–3. doi:10.1016/j.jacc.2015.08.867.

Wu TC, Tashkin DP, Djahed B, Rose JE (1988). Pulmonary hazards of smoking marijuana as compared with tobacco. NEJM. 318(6):347–51.

Zhang Z, Morgenstern H, Spitz MR, Tashkin DP, Yu GP, Marshall JR, et al. (1999). Marijuana use and increased risk of squamous cell carcinoma of the head and neck. Cancer Epidemiol Biomarkers Prev. 8(12):1071–8.

Zhang LR, Morgenstern H, Greenland S, Chang SC, Lazarus P, Teare MD, et al. (2015). Cannabis smoking and lung cancer risk: pooled analysis in the International Lung Cancer Consortium. Int J Cancer. 136(4):894–903.

Zhu K, Levine RS, Brann EA, Hall HI, Caplan LS, Gnepp DR (2002). Case-control study evaluating the homogeneity and heterogeneity of risk factors between sinonasal and nasopharyngeal cancers. Int J Cancer. 99(1):119–23.

Chapter 8

Berk M, Brook S, Trandafir AI (1999). A comparison of olanzapine with haloperidol in cannabis-induced psychotic disorder: a double-blind randomized controlled trial. Int Clin Psychopharmacol. 14(3):177–80.

Coffey C, Carlin JB, Lynskey M, Li N, Patton GC (2003). Adolescent precursors of cannabis dependence: findings from the Victorian Adolescent Health Cohort Study. Brit J Psychiat. 182:330–6.

Crippa JA, Derenusson GN, Chagas MH, Atakan Z, Martín-Santos R, Zuardi AW, et al. (2012). Pharmacological interventions in the treatment of the acute effects of cannabis: a systematic review of literature. Harm Reduct J. 9:7.

Danovitch I, Gorelick DA (2012). State of the art treatments for cannabis dependence. Psychiatr Clin North Am. 35(2):309–26.

EMCDDA (2013). Drug treatment overview for Netherlands [website]. Lisbon: European Monitoring Centre for Drugs and Drug Addiction (http://www.webcitation.org/6S4yjPY59, accessed 15 June 2015).

EMCDDA (2015) Prevention of addict behaviors. Updated and expanded edition on prevention of substance abuse. Lisbon: European Monitoring Centre for Drugs and Drug Addiction (http://www.emcdda.europa.eu/publications/insights/preventing-addictive-behaviours, accessed 05 September 2015.

Faggiano F, Vigna-Taglianti F, Burkhart G, Bohrn K, Cuomo L, Gregori D, et al. (2005). School-based prevention for illicit drugs' use. Cochrane Database Syst Rev. (2):CD003020.

Faggiano F, Vigna-Taglianti F, Burkhart G, Bohrn K, Cuomo L, Gregori D, et al. (2010). The effectiveness of a school-based substance abuse prevention program: 18-Month follow-up of the EU-Dap cluster randomized controlled trial. Drug Alcohol Depend. 108(1–2):56–64.

Faggiano F, Minozzi S, Versino E, Buscemi D (2014). Universal school-based prevention for illicit drug use. Cochrane Database Syst Rev. (12):CD003020. doi: 10.1002/14651858.CD003020.pub3.

Ferri M, Allara E, Bo A, Gasparrini A, Faggiano F (2013). Media campaigns for the prevention of illicit drug use in young people. Cochrane Database Syst Rev. (6):CD009287. doi: 10.1002/14651858.CD009287.pub2.

Fisher BA, Ghuran A, Vadamalai V, Antonios TF. (2005). Cardiovascular complications induced by cannabis smoking: a case report and review of the literature. Emerg Med J. 22:679–80.

Florez-Salamanca L, Secades-Villa R, Budney AJ, Garcia-Rodriguez O, Wang S, Blanco C (2013) Probability and predictors of cannabis use disorders relapse: results of the National Epidemiologic Survey on Alcohol and Related Conditions (NESARC). Drug Alcohol Depend. 132(1–2):127–33 (http://dx.doi.org/10.1016/j.drugalcdep, accessed 05 September 2015).

Foxcroft DR, Tsertsvadze A (2011). Universal family-based prevention programs for alcohol misuse in young people. Cochrane Database Syst Rev. 2011 Sep (9):CD009308.

Foxcroft DF (2014) Can prevention classification be improved by considering the function of prevention? Prev Sci. 15:818–22.

Gates S, McCambridge J, Smith L, Foxcroft D (2006). Interventions for prevention of drug use by young people delivered in non-school settings. Cochrane Database Syst Rev. (1):CD005030.

Hall W, Degenhardt L (2015). High potency cannabis: a risk factor for dependence, poor psychosocial outcomes, and psychosis. BMJ. 350:h1205. doi:10.1136/bmj.h1205.

Hall WD, Pacula RL (2010). Cannabis use and dependence: public health and public policy (reissue of first edition 2003). Cambridge: Cambridge University Press.

Jepson RG, Harris FM, Platt S, Tannahill C (2010) The effectiveness of interventions to change six health behaviours: a review of reviews. BMC Public Health. 10:538.

Jones L, Sumnall H, Witty K, Wareing M, McVeigh J, Bellis M (2006). A review of community-based interventions to reduce substance misuse among vulnerable and disadvantaged young people. Liverpool: National Collaborating Centre for Drug Prevention.

Kosior DA, Filipiak KJ, Stolarz P, Opolski G (2001). Paroxysmal atrial fibrillation following marijuana intoxication: a two-case report of possible association. Int J Cardiol. 78:183–4.

Marshall K, Gowing L, Ali R, Le Foll B (2014). Pharmacotherapies for cannabis dependence. Cochrane Database Syst Rev. (12):CD008940. doi:10.1002/14651858.CD008940.pub2.

McGrath Y, Sumnall H, McVeigh J, Bellis M (2006). Drug use prevention among young people: a review of reviews. London: National Institute for Health and Clinical Excellence (NICE).

Medina-Mora ME (2005). Prevention of substance abuse: a brief overview. World Psychiatry. 4(1):25–30.

Perkonigg A, Goodwin RD, Fiedler A, Behrendt S, Beesdo K, Lieb R, et al. (2008). The natural course of cannabis use, abuse, and dependence during the first decades of life. Addiction. 103:439–49.

Roffman R, Stephens R, editors (2006). Cannabis dependence: its nature, consequences and treatment. Cambridge: Cambridge University Press.

Rubio F, Quintero S, Hernandez A, Fernandez S, Cozar L, Lobato IM, et al. (1993). Flumazenil for coma reversal in children after cannabis. Lancet. 341:1028–9.

Springer JF, Sale E, Hermann J, Sambrano S, Kasim R, Nistler M (2004). Characteristics of effective substance abuse prevention programs for high-risk youth. J Prim Prev. 25:171–219.

Tobler NS, Roona MR, Ochshorn P, Marshall DG, Streke AV, Stackpole KM (2000). School-based adolescent drug prevention programs: 1998 meta-analysis. J Prim Prev. 20:275–336.

Sanders MR (1999). Triple P-Positive Parenting Program: towards an empirically validated multilevel parenting and family support strategy for the prevention of behavior and emotional problems in children. Clin Child Fam Psychol Rev. 2(2):71–90.

WHO (2015), Psychosocial interventions for the management of cannabis dependence (Updated 2015), available at:

http://www.who.int/mental_health/mhgap/evidence/resource/substance_use_q4.pdf?ua=1.